Essential Examination
for Advancing Clinical Practice

Essential Examination for Advancing Clinical Practice

Emma Mellors
Senior Lecturer, Advanced and Specialist Practice – CPD, Faculty of Health Science and Technology, Oxford Brookes University

Vicky MacArthur
Senior Lecturer, Advanced Clinical Practice, Institute of Health, University of Cumbria

© **Scion Publishing Ltd, 2025**

First Edition published in 2025

ISBN 9781914961694

All rights, including for text and data mining (TDM), artificial intelligence (AI) training, and similar technologies, are reserved. No part of this book may be reproduced or transmitted, in any form or by any means, without permission. A CIP catalogue record for this book is available from the British Library.

Scion Publishing Limited

The Old Hayloft, Vantage Business Park, Bloxham Road, Banbury, Oxfordshire OX16 9UX

www.scionpublishing.com

Important Note from the Publisher

The information contained within this book was obtained by Scion Publishing Limited from sources believed by us to be reliable. However, while every effort has been made to ensure its accuracy, no responsibility for loss or injury whatsoever occasioned to any person acting or refraining from action as a result of information contained herein can be accepted by the author or publishers.

Readers should remember that medicine is a constantly evolving science and while the author and publishers have ensured that all dosages, applications and practices are based on current indications, there may be specific practices which differ between communities. You should always follow the guidelines laid down by the manufacturers of specific products and the relevant authorities in the country in which you are practising.

Although every effort has been made to ensure that all owners of copyright material have been acknowledged in this publication, we would be pleased to acknowledge in subsequent reprints or editions any omissions brought to our attention.

Typeset by Evolution Design & Digital Ltd (Kent)
Printed in the UK
Last digit is the print number: 10 9 8 7 6 5 4 3 2 1

CONTENTS

Preface	viii
Introduction	x
How to use this book	xiv
Acknowledgements	xvi
Abbreviations	xvii

System (A–Z)	Why this system?	Examination			Notes
		General inspection	Core examination	Additional examination	
Cardiac	1	2	4	4	6
Ear, nose & throat (ENT)	11	13	14	18	20
Gastrointestinal (GI)	25	26	27	28	31
Musculoskeletal (MSK)	35	36	37		55
Upper limbs			39	44	
Lower limbs			47	50	
Spine			53	54	
General neurological					
General neurological (inc. upper / lower limbs)	67	69	71	73	81
Cranial nerves	89	91	92	98	100

System (A–Z)	Why this system?	Examination			Notes
		General inspection	Core examination	Additional examination	
Peripheral vascular (PVS)	105	106	106	108	110
Respiratory	113	115	117	118	120
Appendices					
Lymph nodes			126		127
General lumps (inc. thyroid, breast, scrotal, hernia)		131	133		138
Skin lesions		145	146		148

PREFACE

This new book is written for the advancing practitioner and aims to underpin a breadth of clinical examination knowledge. It is based on a book originally written to support medical students preparing for undergraduate exams; Alasdair Ruthven's *Essential Examination* rapidly became a trusted resource for a wide range of healthcare professionals seeking to enhance their skills in physical examination. Our version, *for Advancing Clinical Practice*, recognises the diversity of clinicians in roles from nursing to the allied health professions.

Clinicians using this book will be guided to advance their practice by developing a consistent level of high-quality examination skill, in order to flexibly address service user problems arising across all body systems. It is not intended to develop a great depth of examination skills in a particular specialism, nor cover tests requiring additional training, as these are both better supported in specialist texts.

Since its inception in 1948, the NHS has increasingly been required to provide for an ageing population with progressively more complex health needs. Health professionals require development in generalist skills to be able to proactively provide for adult service users with multiple comorbidities. Individual practitioners may have a depth of knowledge related to a particular speciality, but require a breadth of examination skills that they can draw upon when required in order to shorten the service user's journey. Expertise is situational, such that not all clinicians are experts in every situation. Their ability to adapt and apply broad skills to varied situations is what separates levels of skill acquisition for contemporary healthcare demands.

The emphasis in this book is on enhancing an understanding of what is being done and why, to an extent that the reasoning can be verbalised and shared. The history taken from the service user at the start of an assessment is the foundation for this. The crucial role of the history is explicitly emphasised in guiding the clinician's approach to the physical examination. The clinician is encouraged to consider two coinciding agendas: their own objectives and the service user's perspective and needs, to promote mutual understanding as to what is being done and why.

The book offers a 'real world' rational approach to guide and enhance the assessment undertaken by clinicians in advancing practice roles. It also serves as a useful study tool to support preparation for OSCE examinations at postgraduate level.

Emma Mellors and Vicky MacArthur

INTRODUCTION

HISTORY BUILDING APPROACH

Never underestimate what can be uncovered from the service user before any physical examination or investigations are done (Mellors & Macarthur, 2024). Gathering a thorough history can provide up to 80% of the information required to make a diagnosis, but listening carefully also contributes to a person-centred approach (Ospina *et al.*, 2019). *"Listen to the patient, he is telling you the diagnosis"*, is a quote attributed to Sir William Osler, a strong advocate for clinician–patient conversations (Sarasohn-Kahn, 2019).

A narrative approach should be encouraged by asking open questions and allowing the person to tell their story, their way (Mellors & Macarthur, 2024). Useful clues are supplied freely, whilst assisting in the pursuit of a holistic approach (Greenhalgh & Hurwitz, 1999). This could ultimately save time by getting to the crux of what really matters for the person. A practical approach moves the clinician away from taking a history toward building one (Launer, 2018).

Asking follow-up questions to review a person holistically using a thorough review of systems (RoS) approach, moves away from focusing purely on the most obvious body system for the presenting complaint. In this way, useful clues and correlations may be revealed and problems set in a wider context to promote clinical reasoning and understanding of an individual's problems, not just signs and symptoms.

Individuals report problems affecting their lives and can prioritise those which are most disruptive. Constructing a prioritised problem list is a useful way to group a multitude of complaints that make sense to the person having them. Using a timeline, problems can be connected, and elements of a narrative correlated to construct a bigger picture in the context of the whole person. People do not present like textbooks, so not everything will fit into a neat differential diagnosis (DD). There could be more than one disease process but only one illness narrative and there should be room for thinking to evolve as new information and findings come to light (Mellors & Macarthur, 2024). Deal in theories not certainties, as Osler back in the 19th century alluded to:

"If it were not for the great variability among individuals, medicine might as well be a science and not an art" (Olser, cited in Iohom et al., 2004).

Using critical thinking and reasoning, the history given by the service user should be central to guiding the course of the physical examination and subsequent plan of care. Clues from a carefully taken history allow the formulation of theories or DDs that can be tested in the physical examination. In this way, tests are applied with rationale and in partnership with the service user.

In developing examination and consultation skills there should be greater emphasis in partnering with the service user and a focus on explicitly promoting understanding to support their involvement.

A GUIDE TO REVIEW OF SYSTEMS

The premise of advancing practice asks that the practitioner takes a holistic approach to assessment, considering the service user more broadly beyond the obvious presenting complaint. The RoS is an important component of a comprehensive health history that assists in achieving this aim.

The RoS can be focused, extended or complete, based on the acuity of the service user who is presenting and whether this is a first or follow-up visit (Teall et al., 2022). There are two objectives: (1) to obtain additional information about the service user's presenting complaint, and (2) to identify symptoms of potential problems in related systems (Phillips et al., 2017). The RoS is a key part of gathering the clues that will inform the physical examination and plan of care. It may also uncover problems that the service user has overlooked or did not mention, thinking that they weren't relevant to their current health issue.

A RoS is a process of systematic questioning arranged by systems. The questions in the RoS mostly relate to specific symptoms. It should include asking for and documenting any pertinent negative as well as positive findings, but remember to use person-friendly terminology. Any positive symptoms should be investigated using a structured approach similar to that used for interrogation of the presenting complaint, e.g. OLDCARTS (Bickley et al., 2023). The practitioner will then be able to prioritise which systems to follow up in the physical examination.

There are a potentially large number of common or concerning symptoms that may be relevant in each system and examples are shown in the table below. RoS question ideas are indicated in the '**Why this system?**' table at the start of each chapter. This outlines the type of information to seek in order to focus on examining the relevant system.

System	Common or concerning symptoms
Cardiac	Chest pain, palpitations, dyspnoea (orthopnoea/nocturnal).
Eyes, ears, nose, throat	ENT irritation/pain/discharge? Vision changes. Hearing loss. Dysphagia, changes in taste/smell.
Gastrointestinal	Mouth ulcers/teeth/gum problems, nausea/vomiting, appetite change, indigestion, dysphagia, abdominal pain/distension, change in bowel habit, change in colour of stool, unexpected weight loss or gain.
Musculoskeletal	Back pain, neck pain, joint pain/swelling, mobility, falls.
Neurological	Functional/gait/balance/coordination problems, headaches, fits, faints, falls, dizziness/ataxia, tremor, altered sensation, weakness, memory or concentration changes.
Peripheral vascular	Pallor/pain/change in temperature of extremities, claudication, peripheral oedema.
Respiratory	Dyspnoea, cough, sputum (haemoptysis), wheeze, chest pain.
Other	
Genitourinary	Dysuria, urinary frequency, nocturia, haematuria, incontinence.
Female biology	Last menstrual period, irregular/heavy/prolonged menstrual bleeding, vaginal discharge, breast pain/discharge/lumps, contraception, sexual function.
Male biology	Urinary hesitancy/poor stream/terminal dribbling, urethral discharge, erectile dysfunction.
Integumentary	Rashes, lumps, itching, bruising.
Mental health	Energy, sleep, low mood, anxiety, coping/wellbeing.

REFERENCES

Bickley LS, *et al*. (2023) *Bates' Guide to Physical Examination and History Taking*, thirteenth edition. Wolters Kluwer.

Greenhalgh T & Hurwitz B (1999) Narrative based medicine: why study narrative? *British Medical Journal*, 318:48–50.

Iohom G, *et al*. (2004) Principles of pharmacogenetics – implications for the anaesthetist. *British Journal of Anaesthesia*; 93:440–50.

Launer J (2018) *Narrative-Based Practice in Health and Social Care: Conversations Inviting Change*. Routledge.

Mellors E & Macarthur V (2024) How to conduct a clinical consultation in advanced practice. *Nursing Times*, 120:2.

Ospina NS, *et al*. (2019) Eliciting the patient's agenda – secondary analysis of recorded clinical encounters. *Journal of General Internal Medicine*, 34:36–40.

Phillips A, *et al*. (2017). A detailed review of systems: an educational feature. *The Journal for Nurse Practitioners*, 13:681–6.

Sarasohn–Kahn J (2019) Listening to Osler Listening to the Patient – How to Liberate Health Care at Liberation 2019. www.medecision.com/listening-to-osler-listening-to-the-patient, 22 October (accessed 23 February 2023).

Teall AM, *et al*. (eds) (2022) *Evidence-Based Physical Examination Handbook*. Springer Publishing Company.

FURTHER READING

Ball JW & Seidel HM (2019) *Seidel's Physical Examination Handbook*, ninth edition. Elsevier.

Gleadle J (2012) *History and Clinical Examination at a Glance*. John Wiley & Sons.

Ingram S (2017) Taking a comprehensive health history: learning through practice and reflection. *British Journal of Nursing*, 26:1033–7 (https://doi.org/10.12968/bjon.2017.26.18.1033).

Macleod J (2024) *Macleod's Clinical Examination*, 15th edition. Elsevier.

Reno H, *et al*. (2022) *A Guide to Taking a Sexual History*. Centers for Disease Control and Prevention (available at: www.cdc.gov/std/treatment/sexualhistory.pdf).

HOW TO USE THIS BOOK

Each system chapter is split into 3 main sections.

1. WHY THIS SYSTEM?

This section will help you to confirm that you are about to examine an appropriate system. You can use the service user's history, their reported problems and pertinent details to generate theories in the form of potential DDs (please note this list is not exhaustive). Establishing what it is you are looking for, and seeking to test this in the form of DDs early on, will support clarity and organisation of the subsequent examination process. Being able to openly articulate clinical reasoning and justify your examination approach with both the service user and colleagues is an important skill in advancing your practice.

2. EXAMINATION

Examination is the part where you test the likelihood of your theories and aim to **localise** the problem, whilst being mindful of the service user's needs.

A table before each examination prompts you to consider the service user's perspective and supports you to proactively explore any potential concerns with them before you start.

Examination is split into the following sections to encourage a systematic and reasoned approach:

- **General inspection:** this covers commencing the examination process with an initial hands-off inspection.
- **Core examination:** this details components considered essential for the given system and which it is recommended to perform early on in the examination.

- **Additional examination:** this section is where you can use the history, your DDs or core examination findings, to choose additional tests. These tests can support existing findings, explore how widespread a problem is or be used to double-check you are not missing something. It is not necessary to perform all additional tests, but to choose and prioritise based on sound clinical reasoning. Consideration should be made of both time and potential burden of examination on the service user.
- **Conclusion:** this section advises on concluding the examination and next steps in using the findings.

N.B. Please note that the column indicating *'potential findings'* is illustrative and is not intended as an exhaustive list of differential diagnoses.

3. NOTES

Supporting detail and further relevant knowledge can be found here.

ACKNOWLEDGEMENTS

We would like to acknowledge the community of educators and learners at Oxford Brookes University and the University of Cumbria for inspiring our efforts to adapt this resource for the needs of advancing practice in the context of contemporary healthcare demands.

Standing on the shoulders of giants, we acknowledge and thank the author of the original *Essential Examination* book, Alasdair K. B. Ruthven, for allowing us to use his approach and adapt and build on his content.

ABBREVIATIONS

#	fracture		CES	cauda equina syndrome
A&P	anatomy and physiology		CFA	cryptogenic fibrosing alveolitis
AA	abdominal aorta		CFS	chronic fatigue syndrome
AAA	abdominal aortic aneurysm		CHD	congenital heart disease
AAL	anterior axillary line		CLD	chronic liver disease
ABG	arterial blood gas		CLL	chronic lymphoid leukaemia
ABRS	acute bacterial rhinosinusitis		CML	chronic myeloid leukaemia
AC	air conduction		CMT	Charcot–Marie–Tooth disease
ACEi	angiotensin-converting enzyme inhibitor		CNS	central nervous system
ACL	anterior cruciate ligament		COPD	chronic obstructive pulmonary disease
ACS	acute coronary syndrome		CPSP	central post-stroke pain
ACTH	adrenocorticotrophic hormone		CR	chronic rhinosinusitis
ADLs	activities of daily living		CRPS	complex regional pain syndrome
AF	atrial fibrillation		CRT	capillary refill time
ALS	amyotrophic lateral sclerosis		CSF	cerebrospinal fluid
AP	advanced practitioner		CT	computed tomography
APKD	adult polycystic kidney disease		CVA	cerebrovascular accident
AR	aortic regurgitation		CVD	cardiovascular disease
ARS	acute rhinosinusitis		CVS	cardiovascular system
AS	ankylosing spondylitis or aortic stenosis		CXR	chest X-ray
ASIS	anterior superior iliac spine		DD	differential diagnosis
AV	atrioventricular		DDH	developmental dysplasia of the hip
AVN	avascular necrosis		DHS	dynamic hip screw
B12	vitamin B12		DMARD	disease-modifying antirheumatic drug
BC	bone conduction		DIP	distal interphalangeal
BCC	basal cell carcinoma		DIPJ	distal interphalangeal joint
BMI	body mass index		DVT	deep vein thrombosis
BP	blood pressure		EAA	extrinsic allergic alveolitis
BPPV	benign paroxysmal positional vertigo		EBV	Epstein–Barr virus
Ca	cancer		ECG	electrocardiogram
CABG	coronary artery bypass graft		ENT	ear, nose and throat
CAD	coronary artery disease		ER	external rotation
CAM	confusion assessment method		FBC	full blood count
CCF	congestive cardiac failure		FH	family history
CEO	chronic external ophthalmoplegia		FOOSH	fall on outstretched hand

GB	Guillain–Barré syndrome	MCP	metacarpophalangeal
GCA	giant cell arteritis	MDT	multidisciplinary team
GCS	Glasgow coma scale	ME	myalgic encephalomyelitis
GI	gastrointestinal	MGP	Marcus Gunn pupil
GORD	gastro-oesophageal reflux disease	MI	myocardial infarction
HB	heart block	MND	motor neurone disease
HCC	hepatocellular carcinoma	MR	mitral regurgitation
HF	heart failure	MRI	magnetic resonance imaging
HIV	human immunodeficiency virus	MS	mitral stenosis or multiple sclerosis
HM	hepatomegaly	MSK	musculoskeletal
HOCM	hypertrophic obstructive cardiomyopathy	MTP	metatarsophalangeal
HPV	human papillomavirus	NaCl	sodium chloride
HR	heart rate	NOF	neck of femur
HTN	hypertension	NS	nervous system
IBD	inflammatory bowel disease	NSAID	non-steroidal anti-inflammatory drug
IBS	irritable bowel syndrome	OA	osteoarthritis
ICP	intracranial pressure	OE	otitis externa
ICS	intercostal space	OM	otitis media
IDA	iron-deficiency anaemia	P+Ns	pins and needles
IE	infective endocarditis	PAD	peripheral arterial disease
IHD	ischaemic heart disease	PBC	primary biliary cirrhosis
IJV	internal jugular vein	PCA	posterior cerebral artery
INO	internuclear ophthalmoplegia	PCL	posterior cruciate ligament
IP	interphalangeal	PD	Parkinson's disease
IR	internal rotation	PE	pulmonary embolism
IV	intravenous	PEO	progressive external ophthalmoplegia
IVDU	intravenous drug use	PFR	peak flow rate
JVP	jugular venous pressure	PIPJ	proximal interphalangeal joint
LBP	lower back pain	PMH	past medical history
LCL	lateral collateral ligament	PND	paroxysmal nocturnal dyspnoea
LHS	left hand side	PNS	parasympathetic nervous system
LIMA	left internal mammary artery	PR	pulmonary regurgitation
LL	lower limb	PS	pulmonary stenosis
LLQ	left lower quadrant	PSC	primary sclerosing cholangitis
LLSE	left lower sternal edge	PSIS	posterior superior iliac spine
LMN	lower motor neurone	PVD	peripheral vascular disease
LUQ	left upper quadrant	RA	rheumatoid arthritis
LV	left ventricular	RAAS	renin–angiotensin–aldosterone system
LVF	left ventricular failure	RAM	rapid alternating movement
LVH	left ventricular hypertrophy	RAPD	relative afferent pupil defect
MCL	medial collateral ligament (MSK) or mid-clavicular line	RHF	right heart failure

RLQ	right lower quadrant		TB	tuberculosis
ROM	range of movement		TBI	traumatic brain injury
RoS	review of systems		THR	total hip replacement
RR	respiratory rate		TIA	transient ischaemic attack
R-R	radio-radial		TKA	total knee arthroplasty
RS	respiratory system		TM	tympanic membrane
RUQ	right upper quadrant		TMJ	temporomandibular joint
RVF	right ventricular failure		TNF	tumour necrosis factor
Rx	treatment or therapy		TR	tricuspid regurgitation
SAH	subarachnoid haemorrhage		TS	tricuspid stenosis
SBP	spontaneous bacterial peritonitis		UC	ulcerative colitis
SCC	squamous cell carcinoma		UKR	unicompartmental knee replacement
SCDC	subacute combined degeneration of the cord		UL	upper limb
SCI	spinal cord injury		UMN	upper motor neuron
SCLC	small cell lung cancer		URTI	upper respiratory tract infection
SCM	sternocleidomastoid		USS	ultrasound scan
SLE	systemic lupus erythematosus		VEB	ventricular ectopic beat
SOB	shortness of breath		VI	venous insufficiency
SSS	sick sinus syndrome		VSD	ventricular septal defect
SU	service user		VT	ventricular tachycardia
SUFE	slipped upper femoral epiphysis		WCC	white cell count
SVC	superior vena cava		WOB	work of breathing
TAH	total abdominal hysterectomy			

CARDIAC

WHY THIS SYSTEM?

Clues/correlations with history	Cardiac DDs
• Chest pain	ACS, AS, IE, pericarditis
• Shortness of breath	HF, MS, MR, AS, AR, IDA, IE
• Fatigue	HF, MS, MR, AR, IDA, IE
• Palpitations	Arrhythmias (AF, AR, CHD)
• Swelling or oedema	HF, RVF, constrictive pericarditis, DVT, IE
• Fainting	Syncope (cardiomyopathy, valvular disease, aortic dissection, tamponade, pericardial disease)
• Unexplained weight gain	Ascites
• High BMI/FH of hyperlipidaemia/high dietary fat	Hyperlipidaemia
• Smoking history	Increased CVD risk
• FH of young CVD	Increased genetic risk of CVD
• Diagnosis of severe mental illness/learning disability/autism	Increased CVD risk

! BEFORE starting the examination !

Service user perspective: proactively explore any potential concerns beforehand

- Concern for vulnerable exposure: explain the extent of exposure required, reassure about maintaining dignity, offer a chaperone
- Anxiety that this may be cardiac-related and therefore life-threatening: acknowledge and reassure around the need for assessment to make an informed shared decision
- Symptomatic relief prior to examination: oxygen, pain relief
- Minimise position changes if older adult/fatigue/SOB
- May be unable to lie semi-supine if SOB

GENERAL INSPECTION

Component / action	Examine for	DD / potential findings / extra information
Introduction • Wash / gel hands • Introduce yourself, confirm SU, explain examination • Gain informed consent, explain the ability to withdraw or stop the examination • Use draping to expose only as required for each examination step		Consider a chaperone or ask *"Would you like to be supported by someone – is there someone in the waiting room?"*
General appearance	• Unwell / distressed / in pain • Oxygen, fluids & medication	⟶ e.g. GTN spray
Hands • Feel temperature & check capillary refill time • CRT – raise limb above heart level, press on distal phalanx of digit for 5 sec and release (time how long it takes for colour to return – should be <2 sec)	• Peripheral cyanosis • CRT >2 sec • Tendon xanthomata • Osler's nodes & Janeway lesions	⟶ Shock, MI, HF, heart block, VT, tamponade ⟶ PVD, Raynaud's, CCF or with central cyanosis **[see notes 6, 7]** ⟶ Hypercholesterolaemia ⟶ IE
Nails	• Finger clubbing (look closely) • Koilonychia • Splinter haemorrhages • Nailfold infarcts	⟶ IE, cyanotic CHD, atrial myxoma **[see notes 23]** ⟶ IDA ⟶ IE, trauma (e.g. gardening, joinery) ⟶ Vasculitis, SLE
Wrists **Palpate radial pulse for:** • Rate (time over 1 min and compare with other side) • Rhythm • Volume • Character	• Tachycardia • Bradycardia • Irregular **[see notes 9]** • Thready • Bounding • Bisferiens pulse • Slow rising pulse	⟶ CAD, IHD, cardiomyopathy, hypovolaemia, IDA ⟶ SSS, AV block, IHD, cardiomyopathy ⟶ AF **[see notes 10]**, atrial flutter, SSS, IHD, cardiomyopathy ⟶ Shock, pericardial pathology, aortic pathologies, hypovolaemia ⟶ AR, sepsis, AV block ⟶ Mixed AR / AS ⟶ AS
Arms • Measure BP (in both arms if R-R delay)	• Wide pulse pressure • Narrow pulse pressure • Scars	⟶ AR ⟶ AS ⟶ Needle tracks in IV drug use increase risk of IE
Face	• Malar flush	⟶ MS
Eyes (gently pull down lower eyelid)	• Corneal arcus & xanthelasma • Conjunctival pallor	⟶ Hypercholesterolaemia ⟶ Anaemia

CARDIAC

Mouth (use a pen torch)	• Central cyanosis • Poor dentition	→ Lung disease, cardiac shunt, abnormal Hb [see notes 7] → Risk factor for IE
Neck • Palpate carotids to assess pulse character; only ever palpate one side at a time. • Auscultate each in turn for bruits (breath held in expiration with bell)	• Exaggerated pulsation (Corrigan's sign) • Bruit present	→ AR → Carotid stenosis; radiated AS murmur
JVP • SU at 45°, head turned slightly to their left • Use tangential lighting to highlight contours and subtle pulsations • Don't turn head too far – you want neck muscles to relax • Look for double pulsation on right side of neck [see notes 1] • Estimate height above sternal angle in cm • Normally <3–4 cm if raised can measure [see notes 2]	• Prominent IJV extending higher 3-4cm above the sternal angle • Kussmaul's sign (rises with inspiration)	→ [see notes 3] → Tamponade, constrictive pericarditis, restrictive cardiomyopathy

CORE EXAMINATION

Component/action	Examine for	DD / potential findings / extra information
Inspection • For scars and visible heaves • Expose left side of chest, draping right side	• Scars • Visible heave	→ [see notes 5] → Apical (LVH) or parasternal (RVH)
Palpation • Feel for thrills and heaves over each heart valve [see notes 4]: fingertips for heaves, ball of hand for thrills • Apex beat: normally in the 5th intercostal space, midclavicular line; locate & physically count rib spaces, assess character	• Heaves • Thrills • Unable to locate • Tapping • Heaving • Thrusting	→ Right ventricular hypertrophy → Palpable murmur – grade 4 or above by definition → Consider why [see notes 12] → MS → LVH DD [see notes 13] → MR/AR, LVF

Auscultation
• Four primary valve areas [see notes 4]
  ○ Apex (mitral) – [B then D]
  ○ LLSE (tricuspid) – [B then D]
  ○ 2nd left intercostal space (pulmonary) – [D]
  ○ 2nd right intercostal space (aortic) – [D]
Recommended side of stethoscope:
B – Bell
D – Diaphragm
	• S3 [see notes 14]
	• S4 [see notes 14]
	• Murmur
		→ HF, MR, dilated cardiomyopathy
		→ LVH, HTN, AS, hypertrophic cardiomyopathy, IHD
		→ [see notes 16]

ADDITIONAL EXAMINATION

Choose tests according to priority from a range of options (below) based on clinical reasoning – not necessary to do all

Cues from history/DDs/core examination	Component/action	Examine for	DD / potential findings/extra information
Shortness of breath, swelling in ankles, feet or abdomen, sudden unexpected weight gain, chronic cough with white or pink mucus, persistent fatigue, palpitations	Auscultate lungs [see Respiratory]	Crepitations	LVF, RVF
	Palpate ankles [see Peripheral vascular]	Oedema	LVF, RVF [see Peripheral vascular notes]
Raised JVP, anorexia, GI distress, dependent oedema	Abdominal and liver examination [see Gastrointestinal]	Hepatomegaly, ascites	RVF
Osler's nodes, Janeway lesions, finger clubbing, splinter haemorrhages, aortic/mitral regurgitation	Examination of spleen [see Gastrointestinal]	Splenomegaly	IE
Infection or malignancy DD	Axillary lymph node examination [see Appendix for location]	Lymphadenopathy [see Appendix]	[see Appendix]

CARDIAC

CONCLUSION

Component / action	Examine for	DD / potential findings / extra information
Conclusion - Wash / gel hands - Thank SU & allow them to re-dress; check they are OK - Review observation chart (HR, BP, RR, SpO$_2$, temperature) - Decide on next steps with the SU or discuss and follow up once findings reviewed		Return to the aim of the examination – to localise the problem by: - Organising & correlating the history & test findings using clinical reasoning - Gathering sufficient information to allow more confident / directed action - Making a final list of DDs / concerns, in order of priority Action - Put together a reasoned / safe plan to cover all potential problems identified This could include: 1. Request further tests, e.g: haematology, ECG, CXR, echocardiogram 2. Give advice / take appropriate action within scope 3. Make a referral / consult with MDT 4. Use safeguarding / gain a second opinion if any uncertainty 5. Arrange a follow-up

1. How to measure the JVP

With the patient in a semi-recumbent position (at 45°) and their head turned slightly to the left, find the highest point of pulsation of the IJV. Measure the JVP by assessing the vertical distance between the sternal angle (a bony ridge marking the articulation of the second ribs with the sternum) and the top of the pulsation point of the IJV (see *Fig. 1*). Extend a ruler horizontally from the highest point of pulsation. Extend a second ruler vertically from the sternal angle of Louis. Measure the distance from the sternal angle to the point where the two rulers intersect. In healthy individuals, this should be no greater than 3 cm.

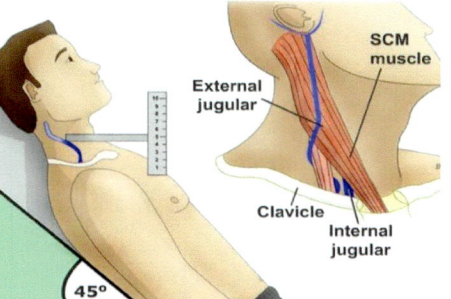

Fig. 1: How to measure the JVP. Reproduced from https://medizzy.com/feed/2859957

2. Features of the JVP (vs. carotid pulse)
- Double pulsation
- Non-palpable
- Obliterated when pressure applied at base of neck
- Height changes with respiration
- Height changes with angle of SU
- Rises with hepatojugular reflux

3. Key JVP abnormalities
- Elevated   RVF, volume overload, PE, constrictive pericarditis
- Elevated with ↓BP   Tension pneumothorax, cardiac tamponade, massive PE, severe asthma
- Elevated & fixed   SVC obstruction

4. Locations where the heart valves are best heard (*Fig. 2*)
- **Aortic valve:** 2nd intercostal space at the right sternal edge
- **Pulmonary valve:** 2nd intercostal space at the left sternal edge
- **Tricuspid valve:** 4th or 5th intercostal space at the lower left sternal edge
- **Mitral valve:** 5th intercostal space in the midclavicular line

Fig. 2: Best places to hear the heart valves. Reproduced from https://courses.lumenlearning.com/suny-ap2/chapter/cardiac-cycle/ (under a CC-BY-4.0 Attribution licence)

CARDIAC NOTES

5. Cardiac surgery scars give you clues during examination
- Midline sternotomy + leg scar = simple CABG most likely, possible valve replacement with CABG
- Midline sternotomy with no leg scar = valve replacement most likely, possible CABG without vein graft (LIMA or radial artery graft only)

6. Differentiating between types of cyanosis
- Pure peripheral cyanosis causes cold blue hands
- Central cyanosis causes blue lips and tongue, and when severe can also cause blue hands (usually warm)

7. DD Central cyanosis (blue lips & tongue)
- Hypoxic lung disease
- Right-to-left cardiac shunt
  - Cyanotic congenital heart disease
  - Eisenmenger's syndrome
- Methaemoglobinaemia
  - Drugs
  - Toxins

8. DD Peripheral cyanosis (blue hands)
- Peripheral vascular disease
- Raynaud's syndrome
- Heart failure
- Shock
- (Central cyanosis when severe)

9. DD Irregularly irregular pulse
- AF
- Ventricular ectopic beats (VEBs)
- Complete HB + variable ventricular escape

To differentiate between AF and VEBs without an ECG you can exercise the SU – this will abolish VEBs but AF will remain

10. Six important causes of AF
- Ischaemic heart disease
- Rheumatic heart disease
- Thyrotoxicosis
- Pneumonia
- PE
- Alcohol

11. Some causes of an absent radial pulse
- Congenital (usually bilateral)
- Arterial embolism (e.g. due to AF)
- Atheroma (usually subclavian)
- Previous arterial line
- Previous coronary angiography
- Cervical rib
- Coarctation of the aorta
- Aortic arch dissection
- Significant hypotension

12. Causes of a non-palpable apex beat
1. Something is between your fingers and the apex
   - Adipose tissue (obese SU)
   - Air (pneumothorax or emphysema)
   - Fluid (pleural or pericardial effusion)
2. The apex is not in its normal position
   - Displaced (usually laterally in LVF)
   - Dextrocardia

CCF = biventricular failure = LVF + RVF

13. DD Heaving apex (LVH)
- Aortic stenosis
- Hypertension
- HOCM
- Coarctation of the aorta

14. Extra heart sounds
3rd heart sound (S3)
- Heard just after S2
- Due to rapid ventricular filling
- May be normal if <30 years old
- Think *volume overload*
- Causes: CCF, MR, AR, large anterior MI

4th heart sound (S4)
- Heard just before S1
- Due to poorly compliant ventricle
- Always abnormal
- Cannot occur in AF (requires atrial systole)
- Think *pressure overload*
- Causes: AS, HTN, HOCM, post-MI fibrosis

15. Causes of cardiac failure
1. Pump failure
   - IHD
   - Cardiomyopathy
   - Constrictive pericarditis
   - Arrhythmia
   - Drugs (negative inotropes)
2. Excessive preload
   - Regurgitant valvular disease (MR/AR)
   - Fluid overload (renal failure, IV fluids)
   - VSD
3. Excessive afterload
   - AS
   - HTN
4. High-output failure (rare)
   - Anaemia
   - Pregnancy
   - Metabolic (hyperthyroidism, Paget's)
5. Isolated RVF
   - Cor pulmonale
   - Primary pulmonary HTN

16. Heart murmurs

		Mitral stenosis	Mitral regurgitation

Aetiology		• Rheumatic heart disease (99%)	• Primary MR (structural)
			  ○ Rheumatic heart disease
			  ○ IE
			  ○ Valve prolapse
			  ○ Papillary muscle rupture (e.g. post-MI)
			  ○ Marfan's
			  ○ SLE
			• Secondary MR (functional)
			  ○ LV dilatation

Presentation		• SOB & fatigue • Pulmonary oedema / haemoptysis • RVF (late)	• SOB & fatigue • Other LVF (orthopnoea, PND)
Features [see notes 17]	T	• Mid-diastolic	• Pansystolic
	I	• 1–4	• 1–6
	P	• Apex	• Apex
	P	• On LHS & with expiration (Bell)	• –
	Q	• Rumbling (low-pitched)	• Blowing
	R	• None	• Axilla
	S	• Opening snap • Tapping apex • AF • Loud 1st heart sound • Mitral facies • Signs of RVF (late)	• 3rd heart sound • Thrusting, displaced apex • Quiet 1st heart sound • Obliterated 2nd heart sound • AF • Audible 'click' in valve prolapse
ECG features		• AF common • P mitrale (bifid P waves)	• AF common • VEBs
CXR features		• Enlarged left atrium • Pulmonary venous congestion	• Cardiomegaly (late) • Cardiac failure [see notes 15]

DD		• Austin Flint (2° AR)
		• Carey Coombs (rheumatic fever)
		• TS (usually rheumatic)
			• VSD (important DD post-MI)
			• TR (usually functional)
			  ○ Pulsatile hepatomegaly
			  ○ Giant V waves in JVP
			• AS (in DD for any systolic murmur)

Treatment		• AF Rx + anticoagulation • Diuretics	• AF Rx + anticoagulation • Diuretics • ACEi (HTN worsens MR)

CARDIAC NOTES

		Aortic stenosis	Aortic regurgitation
Aetiology		• Rheumatic heart disease • Calcified bicuspid valve (age 50–60) • Calcified tricuspid valve (age 70+)	• Rheumatic heart disease • IE • Luetic heart disease (syphilis) • Bicuspid valve • Hypertension • Aortic dissection • Marfan's • RA • Ankylosing spondylitis
Presentation		• SOB • Syncope / pre-syncope • Angina	• SOB & fatigue • Palpitations • (Often asymptomatic)
Features	T	• Ejection systolic	• Early diastolic
	I	• 1–6	• 1–4
	P	• Aortic	• LLSE
	P	• –	• Sitting up & with expiration [Diaphragm]
	Q	• Crescendo–decrescendo	• Breath-like (high-pitched)
	R	• Carotids	• None
	S	• 4th heart sound • Heaving apex • Slow-rising pulse • Narrow pulse pressure • Ejection click • Quiet 2nd heart sound (if severe)	• 3rd heart sound • Thrusting, displaced apex • Collapsing pulse • Wide pulse pressure • Eponymous signs [see notes 21] • Austin Flint murmur (mid-diastolic)
ECG features		• LVH / LV strain pattern	• –
CXR features		• –	• Cardiomegaly • Cardiac failure [see notes 15]
DD		• Aortic sclerosis [see notes 20] • HOCM • PS (usually congenital) • MR (in DD for any systolic murmur)	• PR • Graham Steele (PR 2° pulmonary hypertension)
Treatment		Treat HTN	• Diuretics • Vasodilators

17. System for describing features of a heart murmur

For the non-specialist AP the key features of heart murmurs to note (for the purpose of referral) are T and P1.

It can be difficult to recall the features of a murmur. To help do this, use a method such as the TIPPQRS system. Keep reciting T-I-P-P-Q-R-S to yourself until it comes instantly.

T   Timing
I   Intensity – thrills are rare so generally grade 2 if quiet and grade 3 if loud
P$_1$ Position of stethoscope on precordium where heard loudest
P$_2$ Position of SU when murmur heard loudest – usually only relevant to diastolic murmurs
Q   Quality
R   Radiation
S   Systemic features – other heart sounds, characteristics of the apex beat/pulse, etc.

18. Grading of murmur intensity

- Grade 1   Very faint, just audible by an expert in optimal conditions
- Grade 2   Quiet, just audible by a non-expert in optimal conditions
- Grade 3   Moderately loud
- Grade 4   Loud with palpable thrill
- Grade 5   Very loud with thrill, audible with stethoscope partly off chest
- Grade 6   Very loud with thrill, audible without a stethoscope } Systolic only

19. Stigmata of infective endocarditis

- Changing heart murmurs
- Finger clubbing
- Splinter haemorrhages
- Mild splenomegaly
- Microscopic haematuria
- Eponymous signs (rare!)
  - Osler's nodes on finger pulps
  - Janeway lesions on palms and soles
  - Roth spots on the retina

20. Aortic 'sclerosis'

- *Asymptomatic*
- Does not radiate to carotids
- No slow-rising pulse
- Normal pulse pressure
- 2nd heart sound normal/loud

21. Eponymous signs in AR

- Corrigan's: Exaggerated carotid pulse

- Quincke's: Nailbed pulsation
- De Musset's: Head-nodding
- Duroziez's: Diastolic femoral murmur
- Traube's: 'Pistol shot' femorals

22. Features of finger clubbing

- Increased fluctuance of nailbed
- Loss of nailbed angle
- Increased longitudinal curvature of nail
- Drumsticking

23. DD Finger clubbing

- Cardiovascular disease
  - Cyanotic congenital heart disease
  - Infective endocarditis
  - Atrial myxoma
- Other causes (see also Respiratory and Gastrointestinal)
  - Thyroid acropachy (Graves' disease)
  - Familial

NOTES

EAR, NOSE & THROAT

WHY THIS SYSTEM?

Clues/correlations with history	ENT DDs
• Earache (otalgia)	Acute OM, OE, mastoiditis, trauma/barotrauma, chronic rhinosinusitis, referred pain from teeth/TMJ [see **Cranial nerves – facial function**]
• Sore throat	Pharyngitis (viral or bacterial), tonsillitis, epiglottitis, GORD, rhinosinusitis
• Ear discharge (otorrhoea)	OE, acute/chronic OM with tympanic perforation, cholesteatoma, trauma
• Nose discharge (rhinorrhoea)	Viral URTI, rhinosinusitis, nasal polyps
• Hearing loss/change	Conductive: cerumen impaction, OM with effusion, otosclerosis, tympanic membrane perforation, cholesteatoma Sensorineural: cranial nerve VIII/vestibulocochlear dysfunction: age-related, noise-induced, acoustic neuroma, Ménière's disease, ototoxicity (e.g. aminoglycoside antibiotics [gentamycin], chemotherapy drugs, NSAIDs, loop diuretics [furosemide])
• Tinnitus	Noise-induced, acoustic neuroma, Ménière's disease, ototoxicity, vascular abnormalities, TMJ disorder [see **Cranial nerves – facial function**].
• Vertigo	Peripheral causes (inner ear): BPPV, Ménière's disease, vestibular neuritis or labyrinthitis, acoustic neuroma, perilymph fistula Consider central causes [see **Neurological**], e.g. CVA/TIA, MS, migrainous vertigo, tumours of vestibular pathways
• Swallowing difficulties (dysphagia)	Oropharyngeal causes: pharyngitis/tonsillitis, rhinosinusitis, epiglottitis, retropharyngeal/peritonsillar abscess, oropharyngeal cancer Oesophageal causes: GORD, oesophageal strictures, achalasia, oesophagitis Neurological: bulbar function palsy [see **Cranial nerves**]
• Voice change/hoarseness	Acute laryngitis (usually viral), vocal cord nodules/polyps, laryngeal cancer, GORD, vocal cord paralysis (bulbar function palsy [see **Cranial nerves**], tumour, trauma), thyroid disease
• Smoking history	Increased risk of laryngeal and throat cancer; chronic rhinosinusitis
• Alcohol history	Increased risk of head and neck cancers, particularly oral cavity, larynx and pharynx
• Inhaled recreational drug use	Increased risk of nasal mucosal and septal damage
• Recurrent URTI	Increased risk of rhinosinusitis, OM and tonsillitis
• PMH of GORD	Increased risk of laryngitis, chronic cough, laryngeal cancer
• PMH of HPV infection	Increased risk of oropharyngeal cancer, particularly tonsils and base of tongue
• FH of otosclerosis, Ménière's disease, head and neck cancer	Increased risk of the condition
• Occupational exposure to irritants	Increased risk of rhinosinusitis
• Frequent voice use	Increased risk of laryngitis, vocal cord nodules/polyps

EAR, NOSE & THROAT

BEFORE starting the examination

Service user perspective: proactively explore any potential concerns beforehand

- Fear of discomfort or pain, previous negative experience: explain the procedure in simple terms before starting so that the SU knows what to expect
- Reassure that most procedures are quick and relatively painless; give explicit permission to raise a hand during the procedure to signal discomfort
- Acknowledge anxiety and reassure around the need for assessment to make an informed shared decision
- Feeling of invasiveness due to close physical contact required: use distraction techniques like talking about neutral topics, and short breaks between steps
- Sensitive gag reflex: suggest breathing through the nose during throat exam to reduce gag reflex

EAR, NOSE & THROAT

GENERAL INSPECTION

Component / action	Examine for	DD / potential findings / extra information
Introduction • Wash / gel hands • Introduce yourself, confirm SU, explain examination • Gain informed consent, explain ability to withdraw, stop the examination, decline specific tests or ask questions • Position SU – sitting in chair / on side of bed • Use draping to expose only as required for each examination step		Consider a chaperone or ask "*Would you like to be supported by someone – is there someone in the waiting room?*"
General appearance	• Unwell / distressed / in pain • Hearing aids • Hoarse voice • Stridor • Mouth breathing • Visible otorrhoea / rhinorrhoea	→ Pre-existing hearing deficit can cause ear wax impaction → Laryngitis, vocal cord nodules, laryngeal nerve damage, bulbar function palsy [see **Cranial nerves**] → Partial upper airway obstruction (e.g. epiglottitis, foreign body, vocal cord paralysis) → Nasal obstruction (e.g. adenoid hypertrophy, polyps, deviated septum) → Infection, allergy, trauma
Face	• Asymmetry	→ Nerve dysfunction (e.g. Bell's palsy) → Infection (e.g. OM, rhinosinusitis, cholesteatoma) → Trauma (e.g. facial fractures) → Tumours (benign or malignant, e.g. parotid gland)
Mouth (use a pen torch)	• Cracking or sores on lips • Poor oral hygiene • Gingival bleeding / swelling • Ulceration • Smooth swollen tongue • White patches on tongue / buccal mucosa	→ Nutritional deficiencies, herpes simplex, angular stomatitis → Risk of infections (e.g. tonsillitis, Ludwig's angina) → Vitamin C deficiency, periodontal disease → Trauma, infection (e.g. herpes simplex), malignancy → Glossitis – vitamin B12 or iron deficiency → Candida infection or leukoplakia
Neck	• Asymmetry or swelling	→ Enlarged lymph nodes, infection (e.g. strep throat, scrofula), malignancy (lymphoma, metastases), inflammatory conditions (e.g. SLE) [see **Appendices: lymph nodes & general lumps**] → Thyroid enlargement [see **Appendix: general lumps**]

CORE EXAMINATION – EARS

Component / action	Examine for	DD / potential findings / extra information
Inspection (bilateral) ● Pinna	● Erythema & oedema ● Skin lesions ● Deformity ● Psoriatic plaques (neck & scalp too) ● Gouty tophi	→ OE → Pre-maliganant (actinic keratoses) and malignant (BCC, SCC) [see Appendix: skin lesions] → Acquired (cauliflower ear), congenital (microtia, low-set ears, e.g. Down's or Turner's syndrome) → Plaque psoriasis [see Appendix: skin lesions]; consider MSK examination → Chronic tophaceous gout; consider MSK examination
● External auditory canal ● Character of discharge	● Clear watery ● Purulent ● Blood-tinged ● Thick white / yellow odourless ● Brown or black ● Foreign body	→ Allergy, irritation, CSF leak 2° to trauma / surgery → OM with perforation, OE → Trauma, infection with ulceration, ruptured TM → Cholesteatoma (unilateral) → Excess cerumen, otomycosis, old blood
● Mastoid area	● Erythema & swelling	→ Mastoiditis
Palpation (bilateral) ● Press on tragus ● Gently pull helix ● Palpate mastoid area	● Pain / tenderness	→ Tragus – OE → Helix – OE, trauma, perichondritis → Mastoid – mastoiditis
Test (bilaterally) ● Whisper test – stand behind SU 60 cm away, SU occlude one ear, whisper 3 words; test other ear using different words	● Inability to correctly repeat 2 of 3 words	→ Possible high-frequency hearing loss (sensorineural), occluded external ear canal (e.g. cerumen, infection), noise-induced damage, otosclerosis, Ménière's disease → Cranial nerve VIII / vestibulocochlear dysfunction → If abnormal, use Rinne and Weber to test further [see notes 1]

EAR, NOSE & THROAT

- Examine with otoscope using correct technique [**see notes 4**]
- Bilaterally, examine non-affected ear first
- Ear canal
  - Excessive earwax → Conductive hearing loss [**see notes 2**]
  - Erythema and oedema → OE
  - Discharge → [see **Inspection**]
  - Foreign bodies

- Tympanic membrane
  - Erythema → Inflammation, e.g. OM, myringitis
  - Bulging → Increased middle ear pressure, e.g. OM with effusion
  - Retraction → Reduced middle ear pressure, e.g. Eustachian tube dysfunction secondary to URTI / allergies
  - Absent or distorted light reflex (cone of light) → Bulging with OM
  - Perforation → OM, trauma, cholesteatoma (esp. if in superior TM)
  - Scarring → Tympanosclerosis 2° to OM or grommet insertion

CORE EXAMINATION – NOSE

Component / action	Examine for	DD / potential findings / extra information
Inspection: external surface from front and sides Ask *"Have you noticed any changes in your sense of smell?"*	• Skin changes • Deformities • Report of reduced sense of smell	→ BCC, SCC, keratoacanthoma, cellulitis [**see Appendix: skin lesions**] → Trauma (fracture, dislocation) → Infection, allergy, nasal polyps, chronic rhinosinusitis, olfactory nerve palsy [**see Cranial nerves**]

Palpation
• Nasal bones
• Nasal cartilage
• Sinuses [**see notes 6**]
  ○ frontal – press your thumbs under the bony brow on each side of the nose
  ○ maxillary – press your thumbs under the zygomatic processes
	• Alignment, tenderness, irregularity
	• Alignment, tenderness, inflammation
	• Pain, tenderness
		→ Trauma / fracture, rhinosinusitis
		→ Trauma / fracture, perichondritis
		→ Rhinosinusitis

Test (bilaterally) • Ask SU to occlude nostrils in turn and breathe in	• Occlusion • Congestion	→ Obstruction (e.g. polyps, septal deviation) → Rhinosinusitis, allergy, infection
Examine with otoscope using correct technique [**see notes 5**] • Bilaterally, examine non-affected nostril first • Nasal mucosa • Nasal cavity • Septum • Character of mucus / discharge	• Pale or red membranes • Crusting or scabbing • Polyps • Tumours • Septal haematoma • Deviation, perforation • Clear watery fluid • Purulent (yellow / green) • Blood-tinged • Frank haemorrhage • Foul-smelling unilateral	→ Pale in allergies, red in infections → e.g. chronic rhinosinusitis, dryness → Chronic rhinosinusitis → Squamous cell carcinoma, adenocarcinoma → Nasal or facial trauma → Trauma, cocaine use, chronic use of nasal sprays → Early viral infection, allergic and non-allergic rhinitis, CSF leak 2° to trauma / surgery (often unilateral) → Bacterial infection, e.g. bacterial rhinosinusitis, chronic sinus infection, odontogenic rhinosinusitis (often unilateral) → Nasal / sinus mucosal trauma, neoplasia, fungal infections → Trauma, fungal infections, neoplasia → Chronic rhinosinusitis, nasal polyps / tumours, foreign body

CORE EXAMINATION – THROAT

Component / action	Examine for	DD / potential findings / extra information
Inspection Ask *"Do you have any changes in your swallowing?"*	• Report of difficulty swallowing	→ [See Additional examination]
• Palate	• White slough with underlying erythema • Ulceration • Papillomas – cauliflower-like projections on surface	→ Candidiasis → Trauma, infection (e.g. herpes simplex), malignancy → HPV
• Tonsils	• Enlargement • Asymmetry • Ulceration • Peritonsillar swelling	→ Chronic tonsillar hypertrophy, tonsillitis, glandular fever → Tonsillitis, unilateral tonsilloliths, malignancy → Viral infection (e.g. herpes simplex), malignancy → Quinsy
• Pharyngeal arches	• Inflammation	→ Pharyngitis, glandular fever
• Uvula	• Deviation	→ Quinsy, vagus nerve lesion [see Cranial nerves] (can be normal)
• Floor of mouth	• Swelling / increased prominence of parotid duct ± inflammation • Ulceration	→ Submandibular gland sialolithiasis ± infection → Trauma, infection (e.g. herpes simplex), malignancy

ADDITIONAL EXAMINATION

Choose tests according to priority from a range of options (below) based on clinical reasoning – not necessary to do all

Cues from history/DDs/core examination	Component/action	Examine for	DD / potential findings/extra information
Infection or malignancy DD	**Head and neck lymph node examination** **[see Appendix: lymph nodes for location]**	Lymphadenopathy **[see Appendix: lymph nodes]**	→ **[see Appendix: lymph nodes]**
Difficulty swallowing, globus sensation	Ask the SU to swallow a sip of water to evaluate their swallowing reflex	Signs of choking, coughing, or difficulty swallowing that might indicate dysphagia or aspiration	→ Neurological – bulbar function palsy **[see Cranial nerves]** → Muscular/structural: achalasia, pharyngeal infections → Obstruction: oesophageal stricture, oesophageal tumour, foreign body → Inflammatory conditions: oesophagitis, GORD → Psychogenic dysphagia
Failed whisper test	**Weber test** Purpose: to check for lateralisation of sound How: a 512 Hz tuning fork is struck and placed on the centre of the forehead; ask the SU "*Where do you hear the sound?*"	Abnormal test: sound is not heard equally in both ears	→ Conductive or sensorineural hearing loss **[see notes 1]**
	Rinne test Purpose: to compare air conduction (AC) vs. bone conduction (BC) hearing How: a 512 Hz tuning fork is struck and firmly placed on the mastoid bone (BC) until the SU reports that they can no longer hear it; the tuning fork is then placed near the ear canal (AC); ask the SU if they can hear the sound	Abnormal test: after BC is no longer heard, SU reports that they cannot hear sound once the tuning fork is moved next to ear (BC > AC)	→ Conductive or sensorineural hearing loss **[see notes 1]**

CONCLUSION

Component/action	Examine for	DD / potential findings / extra information
Conclusion - Wash/gel hands - Thank SU, allow them to re-dress; check they are OK - Review observation chart (HR, BP, RR, SpO$_2$, temperature) - Decide on next steps with the SU or discuss & follow up once reviewed findings		Return to the aim of the examination – to localise the problem by: - Organising & correlating the history & test findings using clinical reasoning - Gathering sufficient information to allow more confident/directed action - Making a final list of DDs/concerns, in order of priority Action - Put together a reasoned/safe plan to cover all potential problems identified This could include: 1. Request further tests as appropriate, e.g. FBC, monospot test 2. Give advice/take appropriate action within scope 3. Make a referral/consult with MDT 4. Use safeguarding/gain a second opinion if any uncertainty 5. Arrange a follow-up

1. Hearing tests

The Weber and Rinne tests are both used to assess hearing loss, and they complement each other to help determine the type of hearing impairment (conductive vs. sensorineural). Weber helps identify which ear is affected. Rinne helps determine whether the hearing loss is conductive or sensorineural. Together, they provide a fuller picture of hearing function and the potential cause of hearing loss.

Rinne test	Weber test	Diagnosis
• Air > bone (both ears)	• Central	• Normal (referred to as a positive test)
• Bone > air in one ear (e.g. left)	• Lateralises to same ear (i.e. left)	• Conductive hearing loss in left ear
• Air > bone (both ears)	• Lateralises to one ear (e.g. left)	• Sensorineural loss in right ear
• Bone > air in one ear (e.g. left)	• Lateralises to opposite ear (i.e. right)	• Complete sensorineural deafness in left ear*

* This is because sound is conducted via the skull across to the unaffected right ear when bone conduction is tested, but nothing is heard when air conduction is tested in the left ear.

2. Causes of conductive hearing loss

Outer ear causes:
- Impacted cerumen
- Otitis externa
- Foreign bodies in the ear canal
- Congenital malformations (microtia, atresia)

Middle ear causes:
- Otitis media
- Eustachian tube dysfunction (allergies/infections)
- TM perforation
- Cholesteatoma (unilateral)
- Otosclerosis
- Middle ear tumour

NOTES

3. Causes of sensorineural hearing loss
- Congenital, e.g. genetic disorders, birth complications, infection during pregnancy
- Presbycusis
- Noise-induced hearing loss
- Head trauma
- Medical conditions, e.g. Ménière's disease, acoustic neuroma
- Infections, e.g. meningitis, mumps, measles, herpes
- Ototoxic drugs (e.g. aminoglycoside antibiotics, chemotherapy drugs, NSAIDs, loop diuretics)
- Diabetes
- Stroke

4. Correct use of an otoscope for inspection of the ear
The otoscope is held 'upside down' between your thumb and index finger like a pen. Extend your little finger and place it along the person's cheek so that the otoscope is steady and braced to avoid trauma if the person moves their head unexpectedly; use your opposite hand to gently pull the outer ear up and back on adults to straighten the ear canal (for children under 3, pull the outer ear down and back).

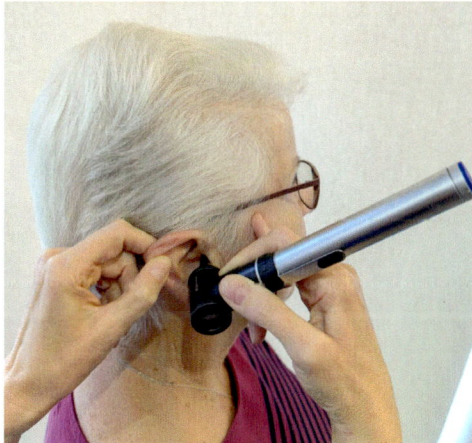

5. Correct use of an otoscope for inspection of the nasal cavity

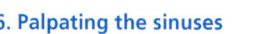

Carefully elevate the tip of the nose with your thumb, insert the tip of the otoscope to examine the nasal cavity.

6. Palpating the sinuses

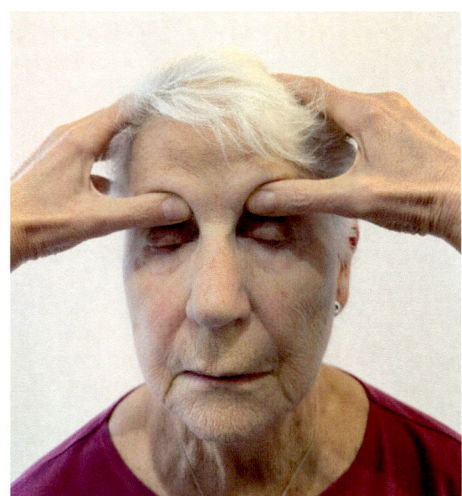
Frontal

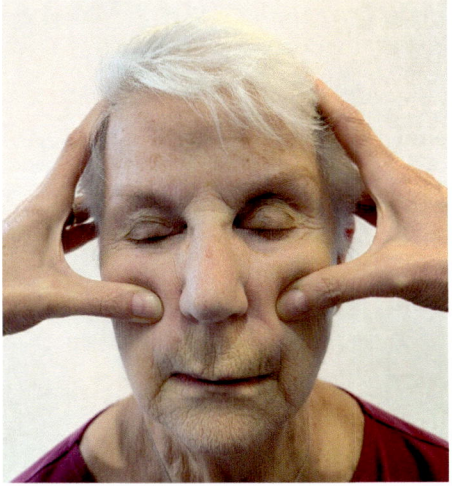
Maxillary

NOTES

7. Rhinosinusitis (the term 'rhinosinusitis' is considered more accurate because sinusitis is almost always accompanied by inflammation of the contiguous nasal mucosa)

Term	Definition	Diagnostic criteria
Acute rhinosinusitis (ARS)	Symptoms resolve within 12 weeks	Sinonasal inflammation lasting <12 weeks and associated with the sudden onset of *at least two* diagnostic symptoms: **Adults** • Nasal blockage/obstruction/congestion or nasal discharge (anterior/posterior nasal drip) • Facial pain/pressure (or headache) • Reduction (or loss) of the sense of smell **Children** • Nasal blockage/obstruction/congestion • Discoloured nasal discharge (anterior/posterior nasal drip) • Cough (daytime and night-time)
Acute viral rhinosinusitis (AVRS)		Symptoms of ARS for less than 10 days
Acute bacterial rhinosinusitis (ABRS)		At least 3 of the following features: • Symptoms for more than 10 days • Discoloured or purulent nasal discharge • Severe localised pain (often unilateral, particularly pain over teeth and jaw) • Fever >38°C • Marked deterioration after an initial milder phase (double sickening)
Chronic rhinosinusitis (CR)	Symptoms last longer than 12 weeks	Sinonasal inflammation lasts ≥12 weeks, with a combination of *at least two* diagnostic symptoms **Adults** • Nasal blockage/obstruction/congestion or nasal discharge (anterior/posterior nasal drip) • Facial pain/pressure (or headache) • Reduction (or loss) of the sense of smell **Children** • Nasal blockage/obstruction/congestion • Discoloured nasal discharge (anterior/posterior nasal drip) • Cough (daytime and night-time) **AND objective evidence of sinonasal inflammation (at least one of the following):** • Mucopurulent mucus, oedema, or polyps on examination • Radiographic evidence of sinonasal inflammation • Endoscopic or CT (computed tomography) evidence of sinonasal inflammation
Recurrent acute rhinosinusitis	4 or more episodes per year with distinct symptom-free intervals	Each episode should reach diagnostic criteria of ARS

From: https://cks.nice.org.uk/topics/sinusitis/

GASTROINTESTINAL

WHY THIS SYSTEM?

Clues/correlations with history	Gastrointestinal DDs
• Acute abdominal pain	Infection/obstruction/trauma/gynae (ectopic)
• Nausea/vomiting	Infection/inflammation/obstruction
• Progressive abdominal pain	Malignancy/inflammation
• Intermittent/episodic chronic abdominal pain	Inflammation/GORD/hernia/gynae (endometriosis/ovarian)
• Bloating	Food intolerance, IBS, constipation, aerophagia, obstruction
• Change in bowel habit	GI malignancy, inflammatory bowel disease (IBD), irritable bowel syndrome (IBS), infection
• Change in colour of stool	Malabsorption, GI bleeding
• Unexplained weight gain/loss	Ascites/malignancy/malabsorption
• Fatigue, SOB	Anaemia due to GI blood loss
• B symptoms*, bleeding/bruising easily	Lymphoma
• Unproductive/dry cough	GORD; consider ENT or Respiratory cause
• High alcohol intake	Chronic liver disease (CLD)
• High BMI/FH of hyperlipidaemia/high dietary fat	Hyperlipidaemia

*B symptoms: fever, drenching night sweats and loss of more than 10% of body weight over 6 months.

! BEFORE starting the examination !

Service user perspective: proactively explore any potential concerns beforehand

- Concern about pain: check for the presence/location of pain and inform SU that you will leave painful quadrant until last in the examination
- Concern for vulnerable exposure: explain the extent of exposure required, reassure about maintaining dignity, offer a chaperone
- Any history of sexual abuse/trauma: trauma-informed approach – put the SU in control
- Give explicit permission to ask for a break/the examination to be stopped if necessary
- Considerations: do they need the toilet? Are they menstruating? Any potential of pregnancy?

GENERAL INSPECTION

Component / action	Examine for	DD / potential findings / extra information
Introduction • Wash / gel hands • Introduce yourself, confirm SU, explain examination • Gain informed consent, explain ability to withdraw, stop the examination, decline specific tests or ask questions • Use draping to expose only as required for each examination step • Position SU: supine at 45°		→ Consider a chaperone or ask *"would you like to be supported by someone – is there someone in the waiting room?"* → Do not lie flat yet
General appearance	• Unwell / distressed / in pain • Oxygen, drips, catheters, medications, drains • Nutritional status / cachexia • Central obesity / peripheral muscle wasting / gynaecomastia / interscapular fat pad (buffalo hump)	→ Wasting due to malabsorption or synthetic liver failure → Long-term steroid Rx, e.g. Crohn's, UC, Cushing's syndrome [**see notes 14 & 15**]
Hands	• Tendon xanthomata • Dupuytren's contracture: *feel* palm for this • Palmar erythema	→ Hyperlipidaemia, PBC, cholestasis → CLD, diabetes, heavy labour, phenytoin, trauma, familial → CLD, pregnancy, hyperthyroidism, RA
Nails	• Finger clubbing (look closely) [**see notes 12**] • Leuconychia • Koilonychia	→ IBD, cirrhosis, lymphoma, coeliac disease [**see notes 13**] → Hypoalbuminaemia (CLD, other causes) → Iron-deficiency anaemia (e.g. GI bleeding)
Wrists • Radial pulse rate: palpate briefly for quick assessment of circulatory status • Assess for flapping tremor: SU extends arms in front with wrists dorsiflexed	• Thready • Bounding • Irregular, jerky downward movement of the hands (asterixis)	→ Hypovolaemia (haemorrhage, dehydration) → Fluid overload, sepsis → Hepatic failure (encephalopathy), respiratory / renal failure
Arms	• Bruising • IVDU marks	→ CLD (due to thrombocytopenia, reduced clotting factors, falls) → Risk of hepatitis B & C
Face	• Cushingoid (moon face, plethora, acne, hirsute) • Parotid enlargement (sialoadenosis)	→ Alcohol excess (alcoholic pseudo-Cushing's, Cushing's syndrome [**see notes 14 & 15**]) → Alcohol excess
Eyes (gently pull down lower eyelid)	• Scleral icterus • Corneal arcus & xanthelasma • Episcleritis / conjunctivitis • Conjunctival pallor	→ Jaundice (implies serum bilirubin >35 µmol/L) → Hyperlipidaemia → Associated with IBD [**see notes 5**] → Anaemia

GASTROINTESTINAL

Mouth (use a pen torch)	• Angular stomatitis & glossitis (large, smooth tongue) → Iron/folate/B12 deficiency • Oral candidiasis → Immunodeficiency • Aphthous ulcers → IBD (especially Crohn's) • Fetor hepaticus (musty, sweet breath odour) → Hepatic failure (mercaptan accumulation)

CORE EXAMINATION

Component/action	Examine for	DD/potential findings/extra information
Inspection • Expose SU from below xiphisternum to mid-thigh briefly: assess femoral area for bulges • Cover to just above pubic symphysis • Observe abdomen from above and tangentially for symmetry, scars, peristaltic movements, contour	• Femoral bulge • Pulsatile bulge • Abdominal distension • Caput medusae (dilated veins from umbilicus outwards) • Scars • Purple striae • Skin lesions	→ Hernia, lymphadenopathy [see **Appendices: General lumps & Lymph nodes**] → Femoral artery aneurysm → The 6 Fs: Fat, Fluid, Flatus, Faeces, Fetus, Fairly big tumour (including polycystic kidneys) → Portal hypertension [see **notes 6**] → Numerous types [see **notes 1**] → Cushing's syndrome [see **notes 14 & 15**] → [see **Appendix: Skin lesions**]
Auscultation • Listen in RLQ with diaphragm of stethoscope until sounds heard or for 2 mins; if no sounds heard move to next quadrant clockwise and repeat until sounds heard	• Hyperactive • Sluggish • Tinkling	→ IBS, IBD, infection → IBD, constipation → Obstruction
Percussion • Assess percussion note for abnormal dullness or tympany • Use tip of middle finger of dominant hand to tap on middle phalanx of middle finger on other hand; elicit a percussion note 2–3 times in each quadrant. Work clockwise and cover whole abdominal area including flanks and around umbilicus. Map out any abnormalities. Consider underlying A&P	• Tympany • Dull • Large dull area • Hypertympanic • Shifting dullness	→ Normal gas → Fluid, faeces → Masses, enlarged organ → Bloating → Ascites [see **notes 2 & 3**]
Palpation Work clockwise starting away from the painful area. Consider underlying A&P. • *"Tell me if I cause you any discomfort"* (watching face is key) • Start furthest away from any tender area • Work round 4 quadrants, palpate lightly with one hand then deeply with two hands	• Tenderness • Guarding • Masses	→ Consider location, intensity and pattern [see **notes 16**] → Peritoneal inflammation → Note location [see **notes 8–11**]

ADDITIONAL EXAMINATION

Choose tests according to priority from a range of options (below) based on clinical reasoning – not necessary to do all

Cues from history / DDs / core examination	Component / action	Examine for	DD / potential findings / extra information
Significant history of alcohol intake, liver DDs	**Liver examination** **Estimate liver size with percussion.** Starting in RLQ, percuss in MCL upwards until the resonance of lung tissue is heard, noting the change in tone from tympany to dullness over the solid liver. Note measurement (6–12cm is normal range). **Feel liver edge with palpation.** Starting in RLQ in the MCL, press deeply and instruct SU to take deep breath to use the diaphragm to move liver downwards. Liver edge will flick under your fingers as it descends. As SU exhales, move your hand 2–3cm upwards and repeat until liver edge is felt, or ribs prevent further progress. If liver is felt, assess for texture and tenderness.	Enlargement Liver edge (in HM): ● Smooth ● Knobbly ● Pulsatile ● Tender	→ Hepatomegaly [see notes 4] → Venous congestion / fatty infiltration → Metastases / cysts → Tricuspid regurgitation → Hepatitis / RHF (capsular pain)
LUQ pain / trauma, B symptoms, symptoms of anaemia, frequent infections, bleeding / bruising, DD portal hypertension	**Spleen examination** **Assess spleen boundaries with percussion:** starting in RLQ near umbilicus, percuss in a diagonal line towards the left lower ribs, listening for the dullness of an enlarged spleen. **Splenic percussion sign:** find the lowest ICS in AAL on the left. Percuss continually while SU inhales and exhales. A change in note from tympany to dullness indicates an enlarged spleen. **Palpate for spleen:** starting in RLQ near umbilicus use same technique as for liver, coordinating breathing with palpation in diagonal line to left lower ribs. As for liver, feel during inspiration (encourages an enlarged spleen to come out from behind ribs) Differentiating between spleen & left kidney [see notes 7]	Splenomegaly	→ Infection (e.g. HIV, TB) → Haematological (e.g. sickle cell) → Cancer (e.g. lymphoma) → Portal hypertension / occlusion → Causes of splenomegaly (past the umbilicus) 　○ Malaria 　○ Myelofibrosis 　○ CML 　○ Infective endocarditis 　○ RA (if low WCC this is Felty's syndrome)

GASTROINTESTINAL

Cushingoid appearance, uraemic complexion (yellowing), pallor, SOB, fatigue, peripheral/abdominal oedema	**Kidney examination** Place left hand behind SU's back below ribs underneath right flank. Place right hand on anterior abdomen below right costal margin. Push hands together as SU takes a deep breath to 'capture' the kidney between them, feeling for size and consistency. Repeat on other side.	Bilateral enlargement Unilateral enlargement	→ APKD, bilateral hydronephrosis, amyloidosis → Hydronephrosis, renal cancer, renal cyst
Severe sudden-onset epigastric pain radiating through to the back, possibly with pulsating mass	**Abdominal aorta examination** Do this *very* briefly – not technically GI but cause of abdominal symptoms. Palpate deeply with two hands above umbilicus to identify pulsation of aorta. Estimate width of aorta (should be less than 3cm).	Enlargement Pulsating mass	→ May indicate an abdominal aortic aneurysm (AAA) or atherosclerosis, signalling a risk of aortic rupture or dissection
SU reports lump or tenderness in head/neck area, B symptoms, infectious/malignancy DD	**Head and neck and axillary lymph node examination** [see **Appendix: Lymph nodes** for location]	Lymphadenopathy [see **Appendix: Lymph nodes**]	→ [see **Appendix: Lymph nodes**]
SU reports lump or tenderness in femoral area, B symptoms, infectious/malignancy DD	**Inguinal lymph node examination** [see **Appendix: Lymph nodes** for location] **Examination of hernia** [see **Appendix: General lumps**]	Lymphadenopathy [see **Appendix: Lymph nodes**] Femoral hernia [see **Appendix: General lumps**] Palpable lump [see **Appendix: General lumps**]	→ [see **Appendix: Lymph nodes**] → [see **Appendix: General lumps**] → Inguinal/femoral hernia [see **Appendix: General lumps**]

CONCLUSION

Component / action	Examine for	DD / potential findings / extra information
Conclusion • Wash / gel hands • Thank SU, allow them to re-dress, check they are OK • Review observations (HR, BP, RR, SpO$_2$, temperature) • Decide on next steps with the SU or discuss & follow up once reviewed findings		Return to the aim of the examination – to localise the problem by: • Organising & correlating the history & test findings using clinical reasoning • Gathering sufficient information to allow more confident / directed action • Making a final list of DDs / concerns, in order of priority **Action** • Put together a reasoned / safe plan to cover all potential problems identified This could include: 1. Request further tests, e.g. haematology, USS, MRI, CT 2. Give advice / take appropriate action within scope 3. Make a referral / consult with MDT 4. Use safeguarding / gain a second opinion where uncertainty 5. Arrange a follow-up

1. Abdominal scars
1. Kocher's (subcostal) – open cholecystectomy
2. Right paramedian laparotomy – various (e.g. pancreatic transplant)
3. Midline laparotomy
4. Nephrectomy
5. Gridiron – appendicectomy
6. Laparoscopic – various (cholecystectomy, appendectomy, gynae procedures)
7. Left paramedian – anterior resection of rectum
8. Pfannenstiel/transverse suprapubic – TAH, Caesarian section

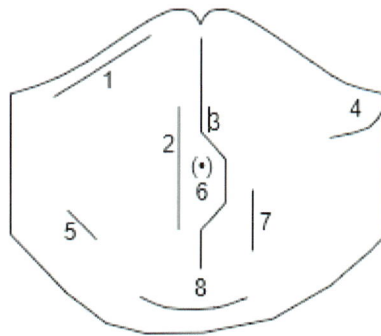

2. Multifactorial aetiology of ascites in CLD
1. Portal hypertension
2. Hypoalbuminaemia
3. Salt & water retention 2° to RAAS activation

3. DD ascites – compare with DD pleural effusion
- **Transudate (protein <30 g/L)**
    - CLD (75% of ascites)
    - RHF
    - Volume overload
    - Hypoalbuminaemia
    - Constrictive pericarditis
- **Exudate (protein >30 g/L)**
    - Infection
        - SBP
        - TB
    - Inflammation
        - Pancreatitis
    - Malignancy
        - Luminal (stomach/colon)
        - Pancreas
        - Liver (primary/metastatic)
        - Ovarian
        - Lymphoma

4. DD hepatomegaly
Remember the categories: 2 Is, 2 Bs & 2 Cs
- Infection
    - Viral hepatitis
    - EBV
    - Malaria
    - Hepatic abscess
- Infiltration
    - Sarcoid
    - Amyloid
    - Fatty liver
    - Haemochromatosis
- Blood-related
    - Lymphoma
    - Leukaemia
    - Myeloproliferative disorders
    - Haemolytic anaemias
- Biliary
    - PBC
    - PSC
- Cancer
    - Primary HCC
    - Metastatic deposits
- Congestion
    - RHF
    - Tricuspid regurgitation
    - Budd–Chiari syndrome

Polycystic hepatomegaly can occur in APKD

5. Extra-intestinal manifestations of IBD
- Finger clubbing
- Mouth ulcers (especially Crohn's)
- Eyes:
  - Episcleritis
  - Conjunctivitis
- Skin:
  - Erythema nodosum
  - Pyoderma gangrenosum
- Joints:
  - Seronegative spondyloarthropathy
- PSC (especially UC)
- Amyloidosis (especially Crohn's)

6. A note on portal hypertension
- Does not *cause* hepatomegaly
- Does cause splenomegaly
- When associated with early hepatic disease (e.g. chronic active hepatitis) which itself causes hepatomegaly, the overall result may be hepatosplenomegaly
- When associated with relatively late hepatic disease (e.g. cirrhosis) which causes a shrunken liver, the overall result is isolated splenomegaly
- Also causes caput medusae, oesophageal varices, gastropathy & ascites

7. Spleen versus left kidney on examination
- You can get your hand over a kidney
- Percussion note is resonant over a kidney
- Kidney is balottable
- Spleen has a notch
- Spleen moves more on respiration

8. DD LLQ mass
- Renal transplant
- Loaded colon
- Diverticular mass
- Colorectal carcinoma
- Ovarian mass/cyst

9. DD RLQ mass
- Renal transplant
- Appendix mass
- Crohn's disease (inflamed, matted small intestine)
- Caecal carcinoma
- Ovarian mass/cyst

10. DD LUQ mass
- Splenomegaly
- Stomach malignancy
- GI malignancy

11. DD RUQ mass
- Enlarged gallbladder
- Hepatomegaly
- GI malignancy

12. Features of finger clubbing
- Increased fluctuance of nailbed
- Loss of nailbed angle
- Increased longitudinal curvature of nail
- Drumsticking

13. DD finger clubbing
- Gastrointestinal disease
  - IBD
  - Hepatic cirrhosis
  - GI lymphoma
  - Coeliac disease
- Other causes [see also Cardiac and Respiratory chapters]
  - Thyroid acropachy (Graves' disease)
  - Familial

NOTES

14. Cushing's syndrome
- Cardiovascular system
  - Hypertension
  - Fluid retention & overload
- Gastrointestinal system
  - Fatty liver
  - Pancreatitis
- Neurological system
  - Euphoria
  - Depression
  - Psychosis
  - Insomnia
- Locomotor system
  - Proximal myopathy
  - Osteoporosis
  - Vertebral wedge fractures
  - Avascular necrosis (e.g. femoral head)
- Immune system
  - Immunosuppression
- Endocrine system
  - Diabetes mellitus
- General cushingoid features
  - Central obesity
  - Muscle wasting in limbs
  - Thin skin
  - Bruising
  - Moon facies
  - Facial plethora
  - Acne
  - Hirsutism
  - Buffalo hump
  - Gynaecomastia
  - Purple abdominal striae

15. Causes of Cushing's syndrome
- High ACTH
  - Pituitary adenoma (Cushing's disease)
  - Ectopic ACTH (e.g. SCLC)
- Low ACTH
  - Adenoma of adrenal cortex
  - Carcinoma of adrenal cortex
  - Iatrogenic (corticosteroid therapy)

NOTES

16. Types of GI pain

Type of pain	Description	Example causes	Clinical features
Visceral	Due to distension of hollow organ or capsule of solid organ	• Peptic ulcer • Gastroenteritis • IBS • Hepatitis/liver enlargement • Pancreatitis • Cholecystitis	• Deep, dull, or aching, difficult to localise • SU may be restless
Parietal	Pain from irritation of the peritoneum	• Appendicitis • Perforated ulcer • Diverticulitis • Acute cholecystitis • Peritonitis	• Severe, sharp, localised, constant – localised to the site of irritation • Aggravated by movement; SU may prefer to lie still
Referred	Felt in more distant site which is innervated at approximately the same spinal level; seems to radiate from initial site as initial pain becomes severe	• Myocardial infarction (MI) • Cholecystitis	• Epigastric pain in MI • Right shoulder or right posterior chest in cholecystitis
Rebound tenderness	Sudden release of pressure applied to abdomen and rapid return of stretched peritoneum causes pain	• Peritonitis	• Pain is worse upon release of deep pressure applied to the abdomen
Involuntary guarding	Reflexive involuntary contraction of abdominal muscles in response to peritoneal irritation	• Peritonitis	• Intense pain on light palpation, abdominal muscles remain tense even when the SU is distracted or reassured
Other causes	Additional causes of abdominal tenderness, including obstruction and vascular issues	• Bowel obstruction • Abdominal aortic aneurysm (AAA)	• Abdominal distension, nausea, vomiting in bowel obstruction • Deep, non-localised tenderness in AAA

NOTES

MUSCULOSKELETAL

WHY THIS SYSTEM?

Clues / correlations with history	MSK DDs
• Most MSK-related diagnoses are accompanied by a primary complaint of pain with varying degrees of cardinal signs: bruising / redness, heat, swelling, pain / tenderness, loss of function	See range of DDs below
• Acute trauma / new-onset pain: location & force of impact are immediate clues to the area involved & severity of damage	Relevant to area of concern: consider full range of DDs from wounds indicating soft tissue damage (superficial or deep) to underlying bony injury
• Acute bony tenderness, deformity or unexpected bony prominence, or hesitancy weight-bearing or moving limb, guarding, accompanied by any cardinal signs	Dislocation, e.g. shoulder / hip / patella; #: open or closed, hairline, non-displaced, displaced, segmental (in 2 places), comminuted (3+ pieces), avulsion (small piece breaks away), compression, greenstick (incomplete in children)
• Joint instability, movement or weight-bearing hesitancy, plus any cardinal signs around joint; acute injury or pattern of chronic tenderness &/or reduced function	Ligament damage: SPrain, degeneration, rupture, e.g. shoulder, knee, ankle
• Localised muscle weakness, muscle fasciculation or hesitancy weight-bearing or moving limb, plus any cardinal signs; acute injury or pattern of chronic tenderness &/ or reduced function	Tendon or muscle damage: STrain, tear, rupture (rare), e.g. shoulder rotator cuff, biceps, hamstring, Achilles
• Localised tenderness in joint region ± history of regular sporting / repetitive activity, esp. wrist/elbow	Stress #, repetitive strain injury, carpal tunnel syndrome, 'tennis elbow' or lateral epicondylitis, 'golfer's elbow' or medial epicondylitis, rotator cuff tendonitis
• Localised tenderness over bony prominence: history may be related to repetitive minor impact, sudden injury, infectious disease or inflammatory disorder	Bursitis, e.g. knee (tibial tuberosity / patella), hip (greater trochanter), elbow (olecranon), shoulder (proximal humerus / acromion)
• Localised joint catching, locking, stiffness or decreased ROM ± cardinal signs; progressive history of joint discomfort or reduced function	Arthritic changes or inflammation of local structures: ligament or articular cartilage damage, e.g. shoulder, hip, meniscus of knee, frozen shoulder or adhesive capsulitis, osteoarthritis
• Exacerbations or progressive history of joint pain alongside cardinal signs, potential muscle weakness / atrophy with decreasing function; associated fatigue or malaise; possible localised bony tenderness, deformity or bony prominence	Arthritic or inflammatory condition, e.g. OA, RA [see notes 1], ankylosing spondylitis (AS), systemic lupus erythematosus (SLE), gout, psoriatic arthritis [see notes 2]
• Widespread pain / pain exacerbations in the absence of trauma, esp. LBP; associated fatigue or malaise; history of repeat investigations / interventions	Chronic pain condition, e.g. fibromyalgia, non-specific LBP
• History of repeated 'accidental' injury, 'clumsiness' or signs of abuse as a cause of injury, especially in vulnerable individuals	Potential abuse
• Risk factors for decreased bone density including gender, age, nutritional status	Osteopenia or osteoporosis, potential stress #

! BEFORE starting the examination !

Service user perspective: proactively explore any potential concerns beforehand

- Concern of pain: check for presence & location of pain & leave painful area until last; give explicit permission to ask that the examination be stopped
- Concern of further injury: e.g. tissue viability or bone #; reassure that looking will enable initial assessment, touch will be cautious & movement avoided as necessary
- Concern for exposure: explain extent of exposure required, reassure about maintaining dignity, offer a chaperone
- Considerations: safety of carrying out specific tests, accuracy of findings if in pain, ways to adapt positions to enable effective testing

GENERAL INSPECTION

Component / action	Examine for	DD / potential findings / extra information
Introduction • Wash / gel hands • Introduce yourself, confirm SU, explain examination • Gain informed consent, explain ability to withdraw, stop the examination, decline specific tests or ask questions • Expose SU to see relevant limb sufficiently; use draping to expose only as required for each examination step • Ensure you know which joint complex or area is painful; ask: "*Can you point to where it is painful?*" & explain "*I would like to compare the affected side with the unaffected side*"		Consider a chaperone or ask "*Would you like to be supported by someone – is there someone in the waiting room?*"

General appearance
• Note age, BMI, general condition
• Note gait & body position
• Note ease of movement & effort required
• Note compensatory movements
 	
• Note facial expression
	• Signs of obesity or being underweight / visible weight loss
	
	• Signs of physical frailty: sarcopenia, increased difficulty & reduced speed of movement
	• Use of mobility aids or using furniture for support
	
	• Signs of pain / discomfort limiting movement:
	  ○ Limping, difficulty weight-bearing
	  ○ Holding a limb to support or protect it
	  ○ Grimacing, laboured, moving hesitantly
		→ Malnutrition: consider malignancy where unintentional weight loss & examine other related systems, e.g. respiratory, GI
		→ Deconditioning, frailty or risk factors for it
		
		→ Ongoing or deteriorating long-term condition, frailty, acute MSK injury or consider neurological cause
		→ Acute injury or painful chronic condition

A NOTE ON MSK EXAMINATION SEQUENCE

A commonly used MSK examination sequence is **LOOK, FEEL, MOVE** for the joint complex of concern (based on DDs) PLUS examination of the joint both ABOVE & BELOW [**see notes 3**]. This is followed by checking neurovascular integrity & any relevant additional examination / special tests for the area of concern. If the area of concern is bigger than a single joint, it may be relevant to expand the examination to multiple joints throughout the upper &/or lower limb & spine. However, it is recommended to start on a focused joint complex guided by DDs.

MUSCULOSKELETAL

CORE EXAMINATION – APPROACH FOR ALL JOINTS

Component/action	Examine for	DD/potential findings/extra information
• Conduct examination using '**look, feel, move**' approach • Examine joint complex above & below area of concern • Examine injured/painful joint complex last		
LOOK • Compare both left & right sides • Anterior, posterior, medial, lateral on & around the area of concern (see each joint below for specifics)	Differences in the skin, muscles, bony structures ('**DRAWS**'): • Deformity • Redness/bruising • Atrophy • Wounds/scars • Swelling/symmetry	→ # or dislocation, tendon or ligament tear, arthritic changes → Acute injury, inflammation → Deconditioning, frailty; consider neurological cause → Acute injury, self-harm/abuse, prior injury/surgery → Inflammation, effusion, infection, acute injury
FEEL • For temperature using back of hands comparing sides • Landmarks on & around the area focusing on the side of concern (see each joint below for appropriate landmarks)	• Heat, swelling • Cold • Deformity • Tenderness • Spasm	→ Inflammation or infection; consider acute septic joint → Potential arterial insufficiency → # or dislocation, tendon or ligament tear, arthritic changes → Acute soft tissue or bony injury, chronic condition → Acute injury or chronic pain

MOVE: compare ROM to the other side if not as expected
• Instruct SU to **actively** move as far as able to go in given movement, to end of their range (see each joint below for required movements)
 	
• Perform movements **passively** where SU struggles or movement is limited, don't force movement
	Reduced ROM and/or pain
	• Reduced ability to perform active movement or in limited range
	
	• Reduced ability to perform passive movement or in limited range
	• Pain on movement or guarding of movement
		→ Bony or soft tissue injury or pain/swelling limiting joint movement; muscular/tendon injury may directly affect ability to perform active ROM
		→ Where concern that reduced active movement is 2° to neurological cause, e.g.
		   ○ Acute injury affecting local neurological integrity
		   ○ Reduced muscle strength in absence of acute injury
		   ○ Associated neck/back pain or spinal injury
		Consider neurological examination, focusing on motor activity tests, e.g. tone, reflexes, power
		→ Increases likelihood of 'true' joint block, e.g. bony, soft tissue or swelling limiting ROM
		→ 2° to acute injury or chronic condition, e.g. chronic pain, OA

Neurovascular integrity
- Check distal to area of concern & compare to other side

Sensation: SU eyes closed, using light touch; "*Say yes when you feel me touch your skin; does that feel normal? Is it the same on both sides?*"
UL [see notes 4]
- Axillary: regimental badge area
- Median: lateral index finger
- Ulnar: medial little finger
- Radial: dorsal 1st interosseous space

LL [see notes 5]
- Peroneal: dorsal foot between hallux & 2nd toe
- Tibial: sole of foot (hallux, little toe, heel)

Vascularity: check for symmetry & grade 0–4+ [see PVS]
- UL: radial pulse & CRT in finger
- LL: dorsalis pedis & posterior tibial pulses, CRT in hallux

- Decreased ability or inability to say when touched
- Abnormal sensations reported

- Absent or thready pulse (graded 0 or 1+)
- CRT ≥3 sec

→ Could indicate compartment syndrome or disrupted nerve conduction due to acute injury, e.g. #, dislocation or swelling
→ Consider decreased or altered sensation 2° to neurological cause (e.g. nerve injury)
→ Perform more extensive sensory testing [see General neurological: additional examination: sensory changes]

→ Compartment syndrome or disrupted blood supply due to acute injury, e.g. # or dislocation
→ Consider decreased circulation 2° to vascular or cardiac cause [see PVS or Cardiac examinations]

MUSCULOSKELETAL

UL CORE EXAMINATION – SPECIFICS FOR EACH JOINT COMPLEX (IN ADDITION TO 'APPROACH FOR ALL JOINTS')

Component/action	Examine for	DD/potential findings/extra information
Shoulder [see notes 6] LOOK: sitting or standing, uncover torso (top off)	• Clavicular deformity • Shoulder looks out of place/displaced humeral head (sunken/forward), ± muscle spasms • Deltoid muscle wasting • Scars • Winged scapula • Axillae (armpit) for obvious abnormality	→ Clavicle # or dislocation → Shoulder dislocation/subluxation [see notes 7] → Deltoid: axillary nerve palsy; consider neurological examination → Arthroscopy, shoulder replacement → Long thoracic nerve palsy
FEEL: landmarks • Sternoclavicular joint, across clavicle to acromioclavicular joint • Acromion on scapula, rest of scapula & its borders • Humeral head, anterior & posterior joint • Long head of biceps	• Clavicular deformity • Humeral head sunken/displaced • Tenderness, swelling • Tenderness	→ Clavicle # or dislocation → Shoulder dislocation/subluxation → Shoulder/subacromial bursitis → Biceps tendonitis, biceps tendon tear/strain
MOVE: standing, useful to do both sides together (start with arms by sides) • Flexion: *"Lift your arms straight up in front of you"* • Extension: *"Move your arms straight behind you"* • ABduction: *"Take your arms out to the sides aiming overhead"* • ADduction: from abduction *"Bring your arms back down to your sides & across your body in front of you"* • Internal rotation (IR): *"Take the back of your hand to the small of your back & move up your back as far as you can go"* • External rotation (ER): *"Aim to take the palm of your hand to the back of your head"*	• Reduced, pain • Reduced, pain, 'painful arc' [see notes 8] • Reduced IR, pain • Reduced ER, pain • Limited ER, painful • Any reduced ROM + pain	→ Biceps tendonitis, biceps tendon or biceps muscle tear/strain → Shoulder impingement/subacromial impingement, rotator cuff syndrome, supraspinatus tendonitis, rotator cuff tendinopathy [see notes 9] → Rotator cuff tendinopathy: weakness/tear/inflammation – degenerative or 2° to acute injury → Rotator cuff tendinopathy: weakness/tear/inflammation – degenerative or 2° to acute injury → Frozen shoulder [see notes 10] → # clavicle/humeral head/humerus; check hand movement: radial nerve palsy (acromion # is rare, consider scapula # in high-impact incidents)

Elbow

Sitting or standing, uncover from shoulders down

LOOK

- Olecranon redness/swelling → Olecranon bursitis, #
- Lateral swelling/redness → Radial head #
- Generalised elbow/forearm swelling, guarding/supporting → Distal humerus #, radial/ulna #
- Raised, red, scaly patches [**see Appendix: Skin lesions**] → Psoriatic plaques: psoriasis (consider psoriatic arthritis)
- Rheumatoid nodules (lumps under skin) → RA
- Cubital fossa/forearm scarring, puncture marks, track marks surrounded by darkened skin, potential abscesses → IV drug use

FEEL: landmarks

- Olecranon (part of ulna) — Tenderness, swelling → Olecranon bursitis, #
- Lateral epicondyle — Tenderness → 'Tennis elbow' or lateral epicondylitis [**see notes 12**]
- Medial epicondyle — Tenderness → 'Golfer's elbow' or medial epicondylitis [**see notes 12**]
- Ulnar nerve behind medial epicondyle — Tenderness, nerve thickening, pain with pressure applied → Ulnar nerve irritation/compression, ulnar nerve entrapment (cubital tunnel syndrome) – check hand function: ulnar nerve palsy

- Radial head & radio-capitellar joint: hold SU's hand in 'shake hand' position, with other hand on lateral epicondyle move downwards into the 'dip' – passively pronate/supinate forearm feeling radial head pivoting under fingers — Pain or stiffness → Radial head #, OA
- Biceps tendon in cubital fossa — Tenderness → Biceps tendinopathy, biceps tendon strain/tear

MOVE

- Flexion: "*Bend your elbows*" — Reduced ± reduced supination, pain → Biceps tendinopathy, biceps tendon strain/tear
- Extension: "*Straighten your elbows*" — Pain, stiffness ± reduced flexion → OA
- Supination/pronation: "*Tuck your elbows into your sides, bend to 90°, turn your palms up to the ceiling & back down*" — Reduced alongside flexion, pain → Biceps tendinopathy, biceps tendon strain/tear, radial head #, OA

- Any reduced ROM + pain → # of any bones in the elbow joint complex: olecranon/ulna/radial head/radius/distal humerus – check hand movement

MUSCULOSKELETAL

Wrist & hand
Sitting, uncover from elbows down, forearms/hands supported
LOOK
- Palms facing down, start at nails, move proximally

- Nail changes, trauma → Systemic illness, injury
  - Pitting, onycholysis → Psoriasis
  - Nailfold infarcts → RA, scleroderma, vasculitis, SLE
  - Finger clubbing, leukonychia, koilonychia → Other system pathology: detailed nail changes related to cardiac, PVS, respiratory, GI DDs [see relevant chapters]
- Fingers
  - Scars → Previous surgery for trauma / OA / RA
  - Swelling / erythema → Synovitis, infection
  - Swan-neck, boutonnière, Z-thumb → RA
  - Spindling → RA, scleroderma
  - Heberden's (DIPJ) / Bouchard's (PIPJ) nodes → OA
- MCP joints
  - Swelling / erythema → Synovitis, infection
  - Ulnar deviation → RA
  - Subluxation / dislocation → RA
- Dorsum
  - Tight, cold, waxy skin with telangiectasia → Scleroderma
  - Interossei wasting / skin 'sinking' between tendons → RA, ulnar nerve palsy; consider neurological examination
  - Rheumatoid nodules → RA
  - Psoriatic plaques [see Appendix: Skin lesions] → Plaque psoriasis
- Wrists
  - Swelling / erythema → Synovitis, infection
  - Radiocarpal subluxation → RA
  - Prominent ulnar styloid → RA

Turn hands over, palms facing up	• Palms	
	○ Scars	→ Dupuytren's release surgery
	○ Thickening of palmar fascia	→ Dupuytren's
	○ Wasting of thenar eminence	→ Median nerve palsy, carpal tunnel syndrome [see notes 13]; consider neurological examination
	○ Wasting of hypothenar eminence	→ Ulnar nerve palsy; consider neurological examination
	○ Palmar erythema	→ RA, hyperthyroidism, pregnancy, CLD; consider GI examination
	• Flexion deformity of fingers	→ Dupuytren's, claw hand
	○ Partial claw: 2nd/3rd digits	→ Median nerve palsy
	○ Partial claw: 4th/5th digits	→ Ulnar nerve palsy
	○ Total claw hand	→ Klumpke's palsy/T1 lesion [see notes 14]; consider neurological examination
	• Wrist scars	→ Carpal tunnel surgery, self-harm
	• Forearms	
	○ Scars	→ Elbow trauma/surgery which may involve ulnar nerve
	○ Rheumatoid nodules	→ RA
	○ Psoriatic plaques [see Appendix: Skin lesions]	→ Plaque psoriasis
FEEL: landmarks Hands: palms down: thumb, fingers & joints • Distal phalanges • DIP joints (not thumb) • Middle phalanges (not thumb) • PIP joints (not thumb) • Interphalangeal joint (thumb only) • Proximal phalanges • MCP joints • Metacarpals	• Bony/joint tenderness/swelling	→ #, synovitis, infection, RA
Hands: palms up • Palmar fascia	• Proximal/thenar eminence tenderness • Thickening	→ Carpal tunnel syndrome [see notes 13] → Dupuytren's
• Wrist joint • General	• Tenderness • Any nodes/nodules	→ Carpal tunnel syndrome [see notes 13] → [see Appendix: General lumps for detailed inspection]

MUSCULOSKELETAL

Wrist: palms down
- Distal radius & ulna
- Wrist joint
- Carpal bones
- Anatomical snuffbox

Tenderness, swelling, deformity	→ Distal radius/ulna #, FOOSH
Tenderness, swelling	→ Scaphoid #, De Quervain's tenosynovitis

MOVE
Fingers: palms up
- Flexion: "*Slowly make fists*"

- Extension: "*Quickly straighten your fingers*"

Fingers: palms down: "*Again make fists*"

- ABduction & ADduction: "*Stretch your fingers apart & then bring them back together*"

Finger scissoring/crossing: abnormal finger cascade	→ Flexor tendon injury, finger deformity
Trigger finger	→ RA, idiopathic tenosynovitis
Loss of valleys between metacarpal heads (knuckles) 2° to MCP joint swelling	→ Synovitis
Reduced/unequal/asymmetric finger ABduction, particularly affecting index finger	→ Ulnar nerve palsy* – check elbow trauma as cause (hand trauma rare)

Thumb:
- Flexion: "*Move tip of thumb to base of little finger*"
- Extension: "*Hand palm down on table, lift up your thumb only*"
- ABduction: "*Palm facing upwards, point your thumb straight up towards your nose*"
- ADduction: "*Bring your thumb next to your index finger*"
- Opposition: "*Touch your thumb to each finger in turn*"

Reduced thumb ABduction	→ Median nerve palsy* – carpal tunnel syndrome [**see notes 13**]
Reduced thumb opposition with little finger	→ Median nerve palsy* – carpal tunnel syndrome [**see notes 13**]

Wrist: palms down
- Extension: "*Bend your wrist up & back*"
- Flexion: "*Bend your wrists towards your forearms*"
- Radial deviation/ulnar deviation: "*Elbows into sides, palms down, move your thumbs towards your wrist* (radial), *then your little fingers towards your wrist*" (ulnar)

- Praying position: palms together, elbows up so wrists fully extended (also reverse Phalen's test)

Unable to perform full wrist extension + MCP joint extension/wrist drop	→ Radial nerve palsy* – check humeral # as cause; C7 radiculopathy, 'Saturday night palsy' [**see General neurological**]

*In absence of acute injury, consider neurological cause (LMN pathology of median, ulnar, radial nerves [**see General neurological examination**])*

Flexion deformity of fingers	→ RA, OA, scleroderma, Dupuytren's
Pain/paraesthesia/numbness in median nerve distribution	→ Carpal tunnel syndrome [**see notes 13**]

UL ADDITIONAL EXAMINATION

Choose tests according to priority from a range of options (below) based on clinical reasoning – not necessary to do all

Cues from history/DDs/core examination	Component/action	Examine for	DD/potential findings/extra information
Shoulder special tests			
Shoulder instability or shoulder pain with history of previous shoulder dislocation	**Shoulder apprehension test** [see fig. 4 in notes 11] • SU supine • Use one hand to stabilise SU's elbow & other hand to support their wrist • Passively Abduct shoulder 90°, flex elbow 90°, externally rotate shoulder	Positive test: 'apprehensive' reaction to this	Shoulder instability/dislocation (glenohumeral joint)
Shoulder impingement or rotator cuff DD, shoulder pain during Abduction, reduced shoulder ROM	**Hawkins' test** [see fig. 5 in notes 11] • SU standing • Use one hand to stabilise SU's elbow & other hand to support their wrist • Passively flex shoulder 90°, flex elbow 90°, internally rotate shoulder	Positive test: pain in shoulder	Supraspinatus tendonitis/tear
Rotator cuff injury/DD, shoulder pain, reduced shoulder ROM	**Jobe's test** [see fig. 6 in notes 11] • SU standing • Say "Straighten your arm out to the side, thumb pointed at floor" • Place hand above SU's elbow – "Keep your arm up, don't let me push it down" – apply resistance downwards	Positive test: pain or difficulty	Supraspinatus (anterosuperior rotator cuff) tendinopathy; weakness/tear/inflammation or impingement syndrome
	Gerber's lift-off test [see fig. 7 in notes 11] • SU standing • Say "Place your hand behind your back, resting the back of your hand on lower back" (mid-lumbar spine) • Stand behind SU & apply light pressure to SU's outward-facing palm • Ask "Push your hand backwards into mine"	Positive test: pain or difficulty	Subscapularis (anteroinferior rotator cuff) tendinopathy; weakness/tear/inflammation
	Resisted external rotation [see fig. 8 in notes 11] • SU standing, arms by sides, elbows flexed to 90° (forearms mid-prone) • Place hands on back of SU hands & ask to "Push out into my hands" – apply resistance to movement	Positive test: pain or difficulty	Teres minor/infraspinatus (posterior rotator cuff) tendinopathy; weakness/tear/inflammation

MUSCULOSKELETAL

Elbow special tests			
'Golfer's elbow' DD or medial epicondyle tenderness	**Resisted wrist flexion test [see fig. 9 in notes 12]** • Ask SU to extend & supinate elbow: "*Straighten your elbow & turn your palm up to ceiling*" • With one hand support elbow & palpate medial epicondyle • With other hand passively extend the wrist (downwards) & hold • Ask SU to try to flex wrist (bend upwards) against you holding it, i.e. against resistance	• Positive test: pain over medial epicondyle →	Medial (flexor) epicondylitis = 'golfer's elbow'
'Tennis elbow' DD or lateral epicondyle tenderness	**Resisted wrist extension (Cozen's) test [see fig. 10 in notes 12]** • Ask SU to extend & pronate elbow & make a fist: "*Straighten your elbow & turn your palm down, then make a fist*" • With one hand support elbow & palpate lateral epicondyle • Ask SU to "*Bend your wrist back (up/backwards) & keep it there*" • With other hand push against the back of SU's hand, making them extend against resistance	• Positive test: pain over lateral epicondyle →	Lateral (extensor) epicondylitis = 'tennis elbow'
Wrist & hand special tests			
Carpal tunnel syndrome DD [see notes 13], median nerve palsy DD	**Phalen's test** • "*Push the backs of your hands together*" (dorsums) • Hold for 30–60 sec (dependent on tolerability) **Tinel's test** • SU palm facing upwards, supported on table • With 2 fingers (index/middle) lightly tap (repeatedly) on median nerve at the wrist (centrally over wrist crease)	• Positive test: pain, paraesthesia, → or numbness in median nerve distribution • Positive test: pain, paraesthesia, → or numbness in median nerve distribution	Carpal tunnel syndrome Carpal tunnel syndrome
Median nerve palsy DD, weak thumb ABduction, reduced gripping/hand function	**Resisted thumb ABduction** • SU palm facing upwards • "*Point your thumb straight up towards your nose*" • With 1 finger resist ABduction by pushing on SU's thumb (palmar aspect) – "*Don't let me push your thumb down*"	• Positive test: weak thumb → ABduction	Median nerve palsy: ABbductor pollicis brevis weakness

Ulnar nerve palsy DD, reduced hand function	**Froment's sign [see fig. 12 in notes 14]** • Ask: "*Hold this piece of paper between your thumb & index finger, trying to keep thumb/finger straight*" • Instruct to grip paper as you pull it away	• Positive test: thumb DIPJ flexes (to compensate for weak ADductor pollicis)	→ Ulnar nerve palsy
	Resisted index finger abduction [see fig. 11 in notes 14] • SU's palm facing downwards • With one hand hold digits 3–5 between your thumb & fingers • With other hand ABduct SU's index finger for them – "*Keep it there*" • With one finger push SU's index finger back towards 3rd finger (resisted ABduction) – "*Don't let me push your finger in*"	• Positive test: weak finger ABduction	→ Ulnar nerve palsy (testing ABduction purely in index finger rather than across all fingers is more sensitive)
Infection or malignancy DD	**Axillary lymph node examination** **[see Appendix: Lymph nodes for location]**	Lymphadenopathy [see **Appendix: Lymph nodes**]	→ [see **Appendix: Lymph nodes**]

MUSCULOSKELETAL

LL CORE EXAMINATION – SPECIFICS FOR EACH JOINT COMPLEX (IN ADDITION TO 'APPROACH FOR ALL JOINTS')

Component/action	Examine for	DD/potential findings/extra information
Hip **LOOK** • Standing, in shorts or pants, from posterior to anterior • Supine on bed, uncover from waist to mid-thighs, look anteriorly	• Scars: anterior, lateral or posterior • Posterior thigh deformity: bulge, swelling, bruising • One leg appearing shorter than the other • Hip held in external rotation • Hip held in flexed or ADducted position	→ Arthroscopy, DHS, THR/arthroplasty (consider possible complications: post-operative infection, dislocation, revision) → Hamstring tear/injury → Fixed flexion/ADduction deformity 2° to OA, # NOF, hip dislocation, previous # femur/tibia, decreased hip flexibility, growth disturbance, e.g. polio, epiphyseal trauma → # NOF: acute or malunion [see notes 15] → OA, joint or bony abnormality
FEEL: landmarks Standing: • PSIS (posteriorly, often visible 'dimples') • Supine on bed: • Iliac crest (posterior to anterior) • ASIS (anteriorly most bony prominences) • Anterior joint line (deep) from ASIS to pubic symphysis • Greater trochanter (flat hand lateral thigh, hip in IR – 'appears')	• Tenderness, esp. over pubic symphysis • Tenderness over greater trochanter	→ Pelvic pain, prior pregnancy, pubic rami # → Trochanteric bursitis (trauma, OA), # NOF
MOVE: Standing or side lying: • Extension: *"With a straight leg, kick heel backwards"* Supine on bed: • Flexion: *"Bring your knee right up to your chest"* • ABduction/ADduction: *"Keeping leg straight, on bed, knee pointing to ceiling, slide it away from the other [AB], then back towards it, can you cross one straight leg over the other [AD]?"* • Rotation: external (ER)/internal (IR): *"Bend your knee, foot resting on the bed, allow knee to fall out to the side [ER], then bring it back towards the other leg, allow knee to roll in as far as possible [IR]"*	• Bending forward to move leg backwards • Back pain ± radiating front thigh pain • Limited abduction ± internal rotation accompanied by pain • Held in ER, apprehension to IR	→ Fixed flexion deformity, OA → Radiculopathy [see notes 18]; consider neurological examination → OA → # NOF, dislocation – anterior (if posterior dislocation likely held in IR)

Knee

LOOK: standing, then sitting or lying, uncover from thighs down

- Scars → Arthroscopy (small), TKA/UKR (large vertical, anterior across joint)
- Swelling → Inflammation, effusion, Baker's cyst
- Fixed flexion → OA, RA, other knee pathology, post TKA
- Asymmetry in thigh circumference → Quadriceps/hamstring wasting 2° to prior injury, surgery
- Bilaterally reduced thigh circumference → Deconditioning, frailty; consider neurological cause
- Varus deformity (bow-legged) → OA, rickets (historically)
- Valgus deformity (knock-kneed) → OA, RA, muscle imbalances

FEEL: landmarks

Sitting or lying, knee flexed to 90°:
- Medial/lateral femoral condyles
- Above, around & on patella
- Patellar tendon down to tibial tuberosity

- Lateral displacement of patella, apprehension → Patellar dislocation
- Visible indentation below patella → Patellar tendon tear
- Tenderness, swelling on/around patella/tibial tuberosity → Bursitis of the knee: supra/pre/infra-patellar (prepatellar = most common) or tibial tuberosity bursitis

- Medial & lateral joint lines, inc. tibial plateau
- Medial/lateral collateral ligaments (M/LCL)

- Asymmetry/reduced joint space, bony abnormality → OA, osteophytes
- Localised tenderness, swelling → M/LCL injury

Leg straight:
- Quadriceps tendon: anterior mid-thigh to patella
- Palpate behind knee

- Deformity: indentation above patella, dropped patella → Quadriceps tendon tear
- Popliteal swelling → Baker's cyst, popliteal aneurysm (pulsatile); consider PVS exam

MOVE: sitting or lying
- Flexion: "*Bring your heel towards your bottom*"
- Extension: "*Straighten your leg out*"

- Locking or catching, inability to extend knee → Meniscus injury/tear: traumatic or degenerative, arthritic changes

- Hyperextension: "*Push the back of your knee into the bed*"
- Straight leg raise: "*Keep your leg straight, raise your heel off the bed*"

- Fixed flexion → Fixed flexion deformity, OA, RA, other knee pathology, post-surgery
- Knee flexion, unable to lift heel, reduced integrity of extensor mechanism – quadriceps to patellar tendon → Quadriceps tendon injury/weakness, patellar tendon injury

MUSCULOSKELETAL

Ankle & foot

LOOK: supported on bed, uncover from knees down

- Shin, ankle, dorsal surface of foot & toes
  - Skin changes: ulceration, flaky, cracks between toes, discolouration, hair loss → Psoriasis, athlete's foot, diabetic foot [see notes 17], Charcot joints [see notes 17] venous / arterial insufficiency; consider neurological or PVS examination
  - Nail changes: onycholysis, trauma → Psoriasis (consider psoriatic arthritis), malnutrition, injury; detailed nail changes related to cardiac, PVS, respiratory, GI DDs [see relevant chapters]
  - Toe deformity, missing toes → Hallux valgus (bunion), mallet / claw / hammer toe, CMT [see notes 17], amputation
  - 1st MTP joint swelling, redness ± ankle → Gout: typical joint involvement 1st MTP joint > ankle > knee > UL

- Plantar surface of foot
  - Normal skin thickening under 1st / 5th MTP joints & heel → Due to normal pressure loading
  - Abnormal callus formation elsewhere → Due to deformity / gait abnormality / abnormal pressure loading

- Heel, Achilles tendon & calf
  - Posterior heel / Achilles tendon inflammation, calf muscle wasting → Achilles injury / degeneration; consider neurological cause

- Examine footwear
  - Orthotics / insoles → Plantar fasciitis, prior foot deformity, pain
  - Asymmetrical wear on soles → Due to long-standing abnormal gait or pressure loading; consider chronic MSK condition or neurological cause

FEEL: landmarks

Supported on bed:
- Medial & lateral malleoli
- Tibiotalar joint (anterior ankle joint line)
- Tarsal bones as a group
- Metatarsals, MTP joints & toes (phalanges)
- Plantar fascia, heel (calcaneus), Achilles tendon & up calf
  - 1st MTP joint heat, swelling, tenderness ± ankle → Gout
  - Tenderness ± calf tightness, difficulty weight-bearing, Achilles tendon thickening → Plantar fasciitis, Achilles or calf muscle strain, tear or rupture, Achilles tendon degeneration

MOVE: on bed

Ankle (tibiotalar) joint:
- Dorsiflexion: "*Pull your toes up towards your shin*"
- Plantarflexion: "*Point your toes away*"
  - Reduced dorsiflexion → Reduced power, foot drop; consider neurological cause
  - Reduced plantarflexion → Achilles or calf muscle strain, tear or rupture, tenderness due to inversion injury (see below)

- Inversion / eversion: stabilise ABOVE ankle joint with 1 hand – "*Move ONLY your foot inwards, then outwards*"
  - Hesitancy, pain or reduced ROM on inversion (replicates injury mechanism) → Ankle inversion injury (sprained ankle) / lateral ligament sprain

Subtalar (talocalcaneal) joint (passive ONLY):
- Inversion / eversion: stabilise ABOVE ankle joint with 1 hand, grasp heel with other hand, invert/evert foot
  - Tenderness on inversion → Ankle inversion injury (sprained ankle) / lateral ligament sprain

Midtarsal / tarsal–metatarsal joint (passive ONLY):
- Inversion / eversion: stabilise directly OVER ankle joint with 1 hand, grasp forefoot with other hand, apply twisting motion between hands
  - Pain/guarding on inversion → Ankle inversion injury (sprained ankle) / lateral ligament sprain

LL ADDITIONAL EXAMINATION

Choose tests according to priority from a range of options (below) based on clinical reasoning – not necessary to do all

Cues from history/DDs/core examination	Component/action	Examine for	DD/potential findings/extra information
Difficulty walking/standing or LL injury/pain	**Simple gait test** ● Ask SU to walk across room, turn & walk back	Expected symmetry, smoothness, step height Expected pattern: heel strike, roll onto toes for 'toe-off' to lift foot & swing leg through ● Antalgic gait, limping, hesitant to weight-bear	Pathology of hip/knee/ankle/foot: localise with specific joint examination according to history
		● Avoiding heel strike	Hindfoot pain, plantar fasciitis
		● Avoiding toe push-off	Achilles injury/instability, calf pain/injury, forefoot pain, plantar fasciitis
		● Reduced plantarflexion/toe push-off	Motor weakness: plantar flexors; consider neurological examination
		● Catching toes or high stepping to clear toes	Foot drop: likely neurological cause – examine
		● Knee: feeling of or actual giving way on weight-bearing	Ligament injury/tear: traumatic or degenerative: ACL, PCL, M/LCL; perform knee special tests for ligament integrity
		● Calf/thigh/buttock/back pain on walking	Neurogenic claudication 2° to lumbar spinal stenosis
		● Waddling gait or 'Trendelenburg' gait, i.e. pelvis dropping side-to-side	# NOF, DDH, SUFE, hip muscle weakness (abductors) 2° to OA or deconditioning; consider neurological, endocrine or infective cause
		● Ataxic, uncoordinated, unbalanced, not smooth or lacking rhythm, unsteady, unsafe, holding self up, leaning to one side, wide stance, high stepping, looking at feet	Consider neurological cause: examine inc. full gait test in neurological examination

MUSCULOSKELETAL

Hip special tests			
Waddling or 'Trendelenburg' gait	**Trendelenburg test** [see figs 14 & 15 in notes 15] • Sit on chair in front of SU • Place hands on SU's iliac crests, thumbs over ASISs • Say: "*Put your hands on my shoulders or arms to support yourself*" • Ask SU to stand on one leg at a time	• Positive test: pelvis tilts downwards/drops on unsupported side & trunk leans in opposite direction to maintain balance →	ABductor instability on standing leg side: ○ 2° to OA, muscle weakness, e.g. deconditioning or nerve root dysfunction/lesion; consider neuro examination (test power) ○ DDH, SUFE
Fixed position of the hip or potential hip OA	**Thomas test** [see fig. 13 in notes 15] • Supine, place one hand in hollow of SU's lumbar spine • Passively flex hip to ROM limit with other hand • Feel that the lumbar lordosis has flattened • Repeat other side	• Positive test: thigh of opposite leg rises up →	Fixed flexion deformity, OA, decreased hip or back flexibility

Knee special tests			
Knee swelling	Knee effusion tests: compare sides **Sweep test** • Leg straight, run hand up medial side of knee 2–3 times • Immediately run hand down lateral side of knee **Patellar test** • Leg straight, from mid-thigh to top of patella, push down front of thigh, hold hand in position • With other hand gently tap over patella	• Positive test: 'bulge' of fluid in medial compartment → • Positive test: floating or bouncing of patella →	Small knee joint effusion (more sensitive than patellar tap) Large knee joint effusion

Knee instability, knee ligament DD	**Ligament integrity tests: [see figs 16–18 in notes 16]** **ACL/PCL drawer tests** • Supine, flex knee to 90°, supported on bed • Sit on SU's foot • Hold behind knee with both hands, thumbs on tibial tuberosity • Stabilising lower tibia with your forearms • Anterior drawer: attempt to pull tibia forwards on the femur • Posterior drawer: attempt to push tibia backwards on the femur **Collateral ligament stress test** • Grasp SU's foot with one hand, support knee with other • Flex knee slightly (approx. 15°) • Stress each side of the knee in turn	• Look from side for posterior sag • Movement without firm endpoint • Movement without firm endpoint • Laxity	→ Lack of PCL integrity → ACL tear/injury → PCL tear/injury → MCL/LCL weakness or injury
Ankle & foot special tests			
Achilles tendon DD or reduced plantarflexion (absent/reduced toe push-off on walking)	**Simmonds' test [see fig. 19 in notes 17]** • SU prone with feet hanging off end of bed, LLs relaxed • Squeeze belly of calf & look for ankle plantarflexion	• Positive test: absence of plantarflexion	→ Achilles tendon tear/rupture
Infection or malignancy DD	**Inguinal lymph node examination [see Appendix: Lymph nodes for location]**	Lymphadenopathy [see Appendix: Lymph nodes]	→ [see Appendix: Lymph nodes]

SPINE CORE EXAMINATION – SPECIFICS FOR EACH JOINT COMPLEX (IN ADDITION TO 'APPROACH FOR ALL JOINTS')

MUSCULOSKELETAL

Component/action	Examine for	DD/potential findings/extra information
Spine LOOK: standing, top off, from front, sides & back	• Discomfort standing, guarding, using support	→ Back pain: acute or chronic cause [see notes 18]; consider GI/PVS cause, e.g. AAA
	• Shoulder, back & gluteal muscle wasting	→ Chronic back pain, RA, deconditioning
	• Increased kyphosis (rounding of shoulders), loss of lordosis	→ AS [see notes 18], osteoporotic #, RA, frailty, postural
	• Exaggerated lordosis	→ Increased abdominal load, obesity, tight hip flexors, postural
	• Scoliosis (S-shaped spine)	→ Idiopathic, neurofibromatosis
FEEL: landmarks Standing		
• Spinous processes (entire length: cervical to lumbar)	• Bony abnormality, tenderness	→ AS, osteoporotic #, RA, neck/back pain related to acute or chronic cause [see notes 18]
• Sacroiliac joints	• Tenderness	→ Sacroiliitis, e.g. AS, pelvic pain, prior pregnancy
• Paraspinal muscles	• Tenderness, spasm	→ Acute injury or chronic pain condition, muscular strain
MOVE: standing Cervical spine:		
• Flexion: "*Put your chin down onto your chest*"	• Neck pain, stiffness, difficulty moving head	→ Related to history: whiplash, repetitive strain, postural fatigue; association with headache, aversion to bright lights, other neurological signs; consider neurological examination
• Extension: "*Look up to the ceiling*"	• Reduced extension	→ AS
• Lateral flexion: "*Try to touch your ear to your shoulder*"		
• Rotation: "*Look over your shoulder*"	• Difficulty turning head	→ Consider cranial nerves examination – spinal accessory (XI) nerve cause
Thoracic/lumbar spine:		
• Flexion: "*Try to touch your toes*" – "*Does this relieve any pain?*"	• Stiffness, hesitancy, pain in any ROM, specific to lumbar ± radiating LL pain	→ Muscular strain, postural, fatigue; back pain ± radiculopathy: acute injury or chronic cause [see notes 18]; consider neurological examination
	• Position of relief for back/LL pain	→ Neurogenic claudication 2° to lumbar spinal stenosis; flexion useful in differentiating from intermittent vascular claudication
• Extension: "*Lean back as far as possible*"	• Reduced extension	→ AS
• Lateral flexion: "*Slide your hand down your leg*"		
• Rotation: stabilise pelvis anteriorly with hands – "*Twist your shoulders round*"		

SPINE ADDITIONAL EXAMINATION

Choose tests according to priority from a range of options (below) based on clinical reasoning – not necessary to do all

	Component / action	Examine for	DD / potential findings / extra information
Spine special tests			
Radiculopathy / sciatica DD, radiating lower back pain down back of LL	**Straight leg raise test [see fig. 20 in notes 18]** • SU supine lying flat • Hold ankle & support front of thigh to keep leg straight • Passively flex hip with leg straight • Normally 90° of pain-free passive hip flexion should be possible	• Positive test: back pain radiating down posterior leg	→ L5/S1 nerve root compression / sciatic nerve irritation / sciatica; consider neurological examination
Radiculopathy DD, radiating lower back pain down front of thigh	**Femoral stretch test [see fig. 21 in notes 18]** • SU lying on front • Hold thigh & ankle, keep leg straight • Passively extend hip	• Positive test: back pain radiating down anterior leg	→ L4 nerve root compression; consider neurological examination

CONCLUSION

Component / action	Examine for	DD / potential findings / extra information
Conclusion • Wash / gel hands • Thank SU, allow them to re-dress, check they are OK • Review observations (HR, BP, RR, SpO$_2$, temperature) • Decide on next steps with the SU or discuss & follow up once reviewed findings		Return to the aim of the examination – to localise the problem by: • Organising & correlating the history & test findings using clinical reasoning • Gathering sufficient information to allow more confident / directed action • Making a final list of DDs / concerns, in order of priority **Action** • Put together a reasoned / safe plan to cover all potential problems identified This could include: 1. Request further tests, e.g. imaging 2. Give advice / take appropriate action within scope, e.g. dressings / supports, advice on activity levels / managing inflammation / pain 3. Make a referral / consult with MDT, e.g. orthopaedics, physio / occupational therapies, frailty team, pain specialist 4. Use safeguarding / gain a second opinion where uncertainty 5. Arrange a follow-up

1. Rheumatoid arthritis

Common presentation of RA: a symmetrical, deforming polyarthropathy affecting the small joints of the hands in a rheumatoid pattern; the most common differentials for this clinical picture are RA & psoriatic arthropathy.

RA statistics
- 3 females : 1 male
- Peak prevalence age 30–50
- 70% seropositive (as is 5% of general population)
  - Rheumatoid factor +ve (IgM against self-IgG)
  - Often have nodules
  - Extra-articular features
  - Progressive disease
- 20% of all RA SUs have nodules
- 50% HLA-DR4 +ve (severe, erosive disease)

Features of active RA
- Inflamed joints
  - Red
  - Hot
  - Swollen
  - Tender
- Pain on passive movement
- Increased duration of morning stiffness
- Raised ESR
- Anaemia [see below]

Extra-articular features of RA
- General: malaise, lethargy, low-grade fever, weight loss
- CVS: pericarditis, pericardial effusion
- RS: nodules, pleural effusion, pulmonary fibrosis, pneumoconiosis (Caplan's syndrome)
- Genitourinary system: renal amyloid
- NS: polyneuropathy, mononeuritis multiplex, carpal tunnel, atlanto-axial subluxation
- Eyes: scleritis, episcleritis, keratoconjunctivitis sicca, Sjögren's syndrome
- Blood: anaemia [see below], thrombocytosis, ↓WCC (Felty's syndrome = ↓WCC + splenomegaly + RA)

Multifactorial aetiology of anaemia in RA
- Anaemia of chronic disease
- Iron-deficiency anaemia secondary to NSAID-induced gastritis/peptic ulcer
- Aplastic anaemia secondary to DMARD
- Macrocytic anaemia secondary to methotrexate (folate metabolism)
- Pernicious anaemia (associated with RA)

Disease-modifying antirheumatic drugs (DMARDs) & key side-effects
- All DMARDs
  - Immunocompromise & infection
  - Marrow suppression
  - Hepatotoxicity
  - Rash
  - GI upset (especially nausea & oral ulcers)
- Methotrexate
  - Pneumonitis & pulmonary fibrosis [see **Respiratory notes 2**]
  - Megaloblastic anaemia
- Hydroxychloroquine
  - Retinopathy
- Sulfasalazine
  - Oligospermia
- IM Gold
  - Nephrotic syndrome
- Penicillamine
  - Nephrotic syndrome
  - Altered taste
  - Myasthenia gravis-like syndrome
- Ciclosporin
  - Renal impairment
  - HTN
  - Gum hypertrophy
- Leflunomide
- Azathioprine
- Biological (e.g. adalimumab, etanercept, infliximab)

Sjögren's syndrome
- May occur independently
- May be associated with RA/SLE/scleroderma
- Features
  - Dry eyes (keratoconjunctivitis sicca)
  - Dry mouth (xerostomia)
  - Parotid gland enlargement

2. Psoriatic arthritis

Psoriatic arthropathy
- Affects 10% of SUs with psoriasis
- In 75% skin features present before arthropathy
- In 20% skin features present after arthropathy
- In 5% no skin features will ever appear

Presentations of psoriatic arthropathy
- Asymmetrical oligoarthritis
  - Mainly hands & feet (dactylitis)
  - Sometimes larger joints
- Lone DIP disease
- Rheumatoid pattern
- Arthritis mutilans
- Sacroiliitis

3. Joint complex above & below table

Joint complex of concern	Joint complex above	Joint complex below
Upper limb		
Shoulder	Cervical spine	Elbow
Elbow	Shoulder	Wrist & hand
Wrist	Elbow	Hand
Hand	Wrist	None
Lower limb		
Hip	Thoracic / lumbar spine	Knee
Knee	Hip	Ankle & foot
Ankle	Knee	Foot
Foot	Ankle	None
Spine		
Cervical spine	None	Thoracic / lumbar spine
Thoracic / lumbar spine	Cervical spine	Hip

NOTES

4. Sensory innervation of the hands

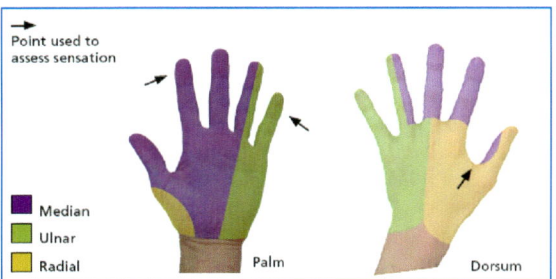

Fig. 1. Sensory innervation of the left hand by the peripheral nerves

5. Sensory innervation of the feet

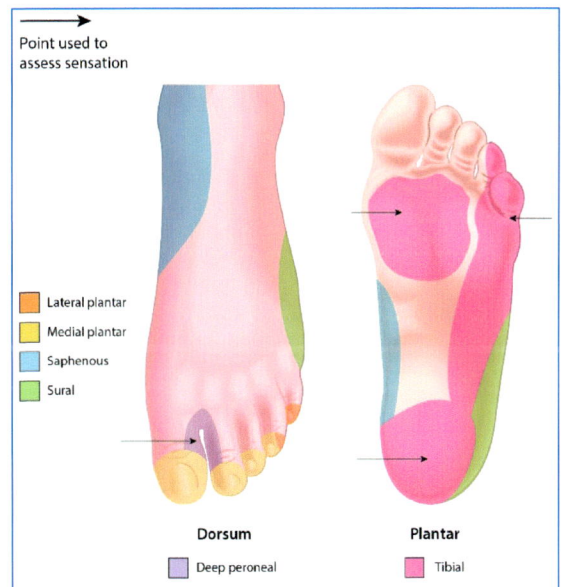

Fig. 2. Sensory innervation of the left foot by the peripheral nerves

6. Common shoulder pathology
1. Instability
   - Usually young SU
   - Previous dislocation(s)
   - Shoulder apprehension test
2. Impingement syndrome
   - Usually middle-aged SU
   - Hawkins' test
3. Rotator cuff tear
   - Usually older SU
   - Test components of rotator cuff
     - Supraspinatus
       – Anterosuperior cuff
       – Jobe's test
     - Subscapularis
       – Anteroinferior cuff
       – Gerber's lift-off test
     - Teres minor & infraspinatus
       – Posterior cuff
       – Resisted external shoulder rotation

7. Complications of anterior dislocation of shoulder (95% of dislocations are anterior)
- Axillary nerve damage
- Brachial plexus/other nerve damage
- Axillary artery damage
- Associated # (30% of cases)
  - Humeral head
  - Clavicle
  - Acromion
- Recurrent shoulder dislocation
- Anatomical lesion
  - Bankart
  - Hill–Sachs
- Rotator cuff injury

8. Shoulder abduction 'painful arc'

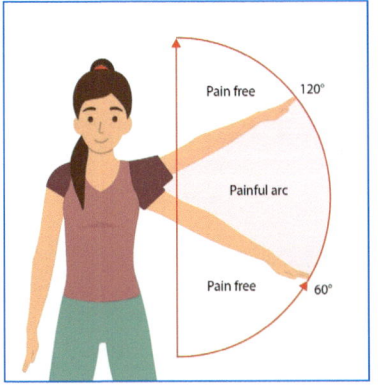

Fig. 3: The painful arc in shoulder ABduction.

9. Impingement syndrome
- Also known as painful arc syndrome
- Underlying pathology is supraspinatus tendonitis
- Painful arc
  - Classical sign of supraspinatus tendonitis
  - Pain during shoulder ABduction between 60° & 120°
  - Due to 'impingement' of the underside of the acromion on the inflamed tendon
- Positive Hawkins' test
  - Arm flexed to 90°
  - Elbow flexed to 90°
  - Shoulder internally rotated, pushing supraspinatus tendon up against acromion
  - Forcing further internal rotation causes pain if tendon is inflamed
  - (Note: Jobe's test for supraspinatus weakness/tear may also cause pain)

10. Frozen shoulder
- Adhesive capsulitis of glenohumeral joint
- Most commonly affects ages 40–65
- Can occur
  - Spontaneously
  - Following rotator cuff injury
  - Following immobility (e.g. stroke)
- Diabetes & thyroid disease are risk factors
- Phases
  - Freezing phase
    - gradual onset of shoulder pain & stiffness
    - 2–9 months
  - Frozen phase
    - pain subsides but stiffness remains
    - external rotation usually very limited
    - 4–12 months
  - Thawing phase
    - gradual return of movement
    - recovery may be incomplete
    - 1–3 years

11. Shoulder test notes

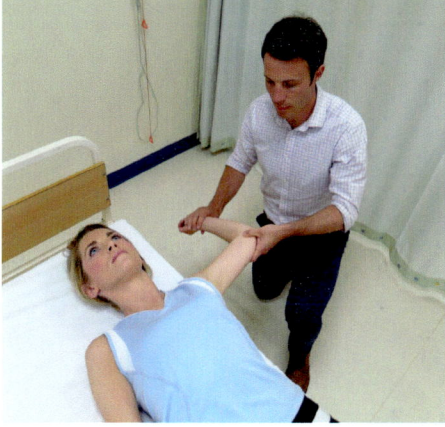

Fig. 4. Shoulder apprehension test. Shoulder instability (usually previous dislocation).

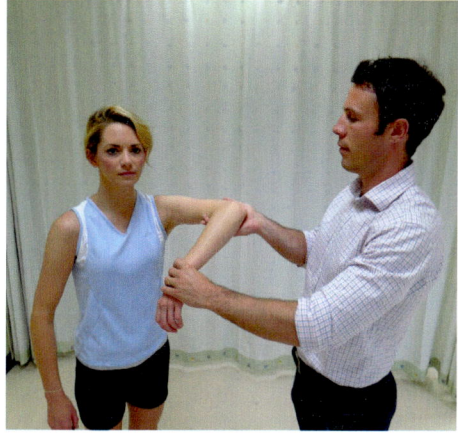

Fig. 5. Hawkins' test. Impingement syndrome.

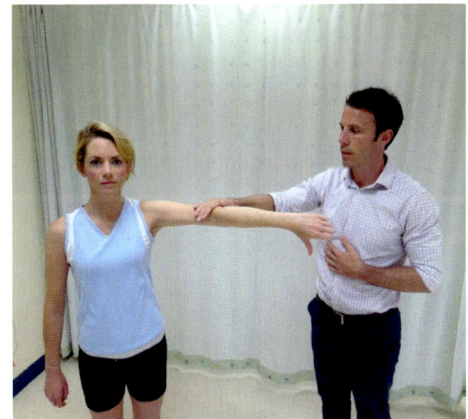

Fig. 6. Jobe's test. Supraspinatus pathology.

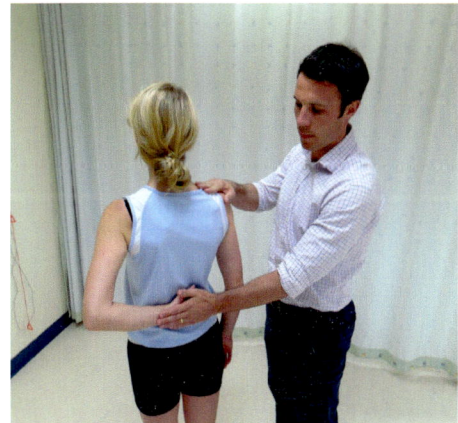

Fig. 7. Gerber's lift-off test. Subscapularis pathology.

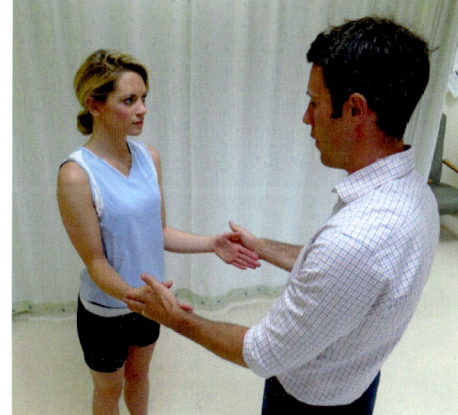

Fig. 8. Resisted external rotation. Teres minor/infraspinatus pathology.

12. Elbow & wrist notes

Tennis & golfer's elbow
- Tennis elbow = extensor epicondylitis (lateral epicondyle)
- Golfer's elbow = flexor epicondylitis (medial epicondyle)
- Gradual onset of lateral (tennis)/medial (golfer's) elbow pain, often radiating into forearm
- Peak incidence age 40–50
- Tennis elbow is 5 times more common than golfer's elbow
- Both are caused by repetitive, often strenuous activity
  - Sports (e.g. tennis/golf... either sport can cause either condition)
  - Heavy lifting
  - DIY
  - Gardening
  - Computer use
- Conservative management
  - Avoid activities that exacerbate symptoms
  - Analgesia & topical NSAIDs
  - Corticosteroid injections
  - Physiotherapy
  - Use of a forearm band orthosis
- Surgical tendon release is rarely required

NOTES

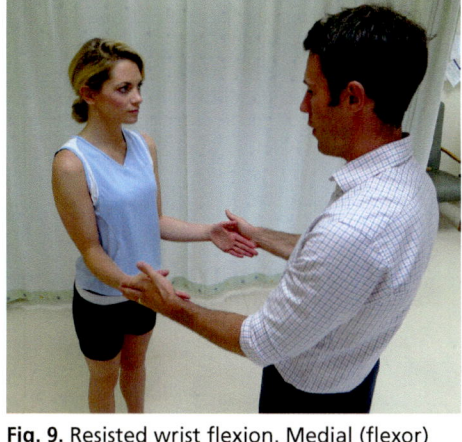

Fig. 9. Resisted wrist flexion. Medial (flexor) epicondylitis = 'golfer's elbow'.

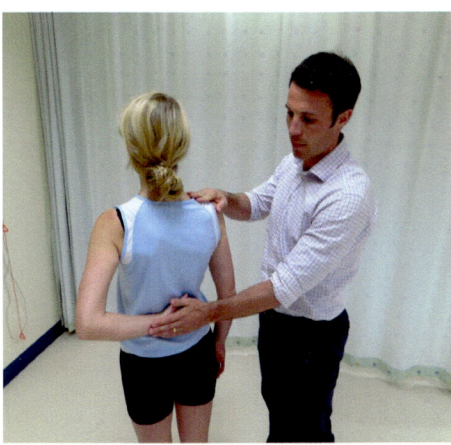

Fig. 10. Resisted wrist extension. Lateral (extensor) epicondylitis = 'tennis elbow'.

13. DD carpal tunnel syndrome
- Idiopathic (majority of cases)
- Mechanical: repetitive strain/compression/entrapment/injury/arthritic/obesity
- Inflammatory: irritation/strain/arthritic/obesity
- Pregnancy
- RA
- Hypothyroid
- Diabetes
- Acromegaly

14. Hand notes
T1 lesion
- Aetiology
  - Cervical spondylosis
  - Pancoast tumour
  - Plexus trauma/birth injury (Klumpke's palsy)
- Clinical features
  - Total claw hand (all lumbricals lost)
  - Wasting of small muscles in hand
  - Pain/sensory loss in medial forearm
  - Horner's syndrome may co-exist

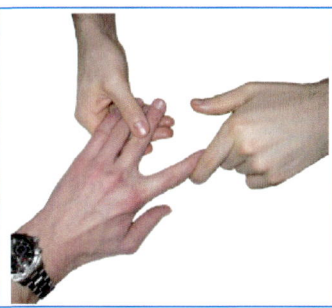

Fig. 11. Assessment of finger ABduction (ulnar nerve).

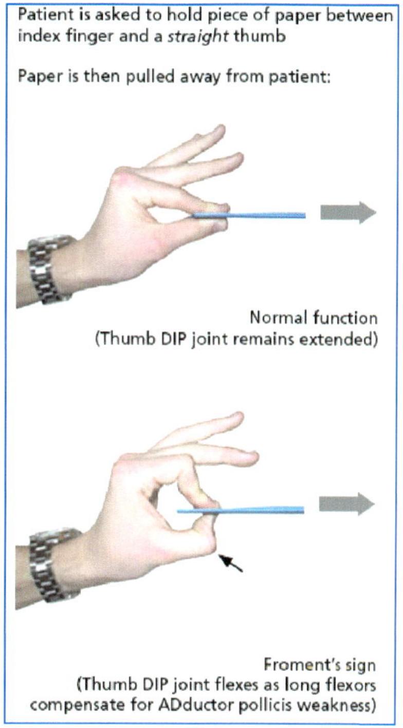

Fig. 12. Froment's sign (ulnar palsy).

15. Hip notes

Neck of femur #

- Usually elderly, osteoporotic SU following low-velocity fall onto hip
- Blood supply to the femoral head
  1. Cervical vessels running in the joint capsule retinaculum (*main supply*)
  2. Intramedullary vessels in the femoral neck
  3. Vessels of the ligamentum teres (negligible contribution, often non-existent)
- Undisplaced intracapsular #
  - Likely disruption of intramedullary vessels but preservation of cervical vessels
  - Low risk of avascular necrosis (AVN) of the femoral head
  - Usually fixed with a dynamic hip screw or cannulated screws

- Displaced intracapsular #
  - Inevitable interruption of intramedullary vessels & likely disruption of cervical vessels
  - High risk of AVN
  - Usually treated with hemiarthroplasty (older patients) or total hip arthroplasty (younger patients with fewer comorbidities & high functional demand)
  - Fixation (e.g. DHS) is reserved for young patients (generally <50 years old) where it is preferable to avoid arthroplasty & accept the risk of AVN

- Extracapsular #
  - Little interruption to blood supply of femoral head
  - Low risk of AVN
  - Intertrochanteric #s are fixed with a DHS
  - Subtrochanteric #s are fixed with a cephalomedullary nail (intramedullary femoral nail with supplemental screws into the femoral head)

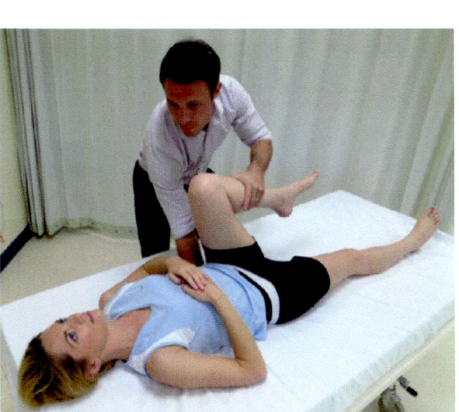

Fig. 13. Thomas test. Feel for flattening of lumbar lordosis & look for opposite thigh rising up due to a fixed flexion deformity of that hip. It is also important to watch the patient's face to ensure you don't cause pain.

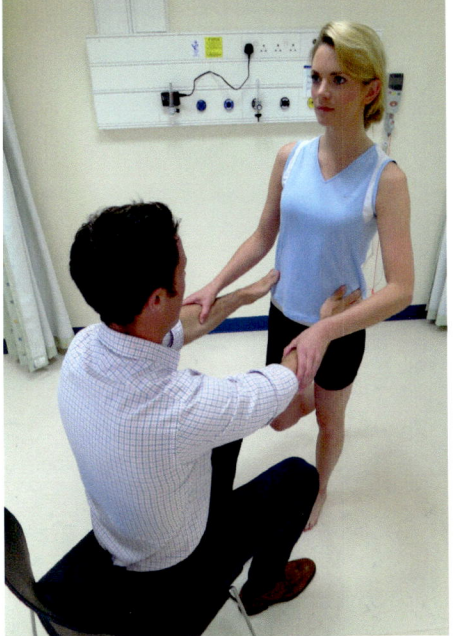

Fig. 14. Trendelenburg test. Negative (normal) result – pelvis tilts up on the unsupported side (right side here).

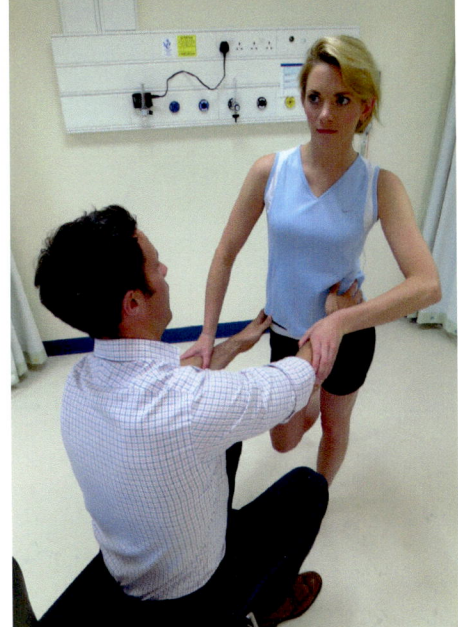

Fig. 15. Trendelenburg test. Positive (abnormal) result due to hip ABductor instability – pelvis drops down on the unsupported (right) side & trunk leans to the opposite (left) side to keep balance.

16. Knee notes

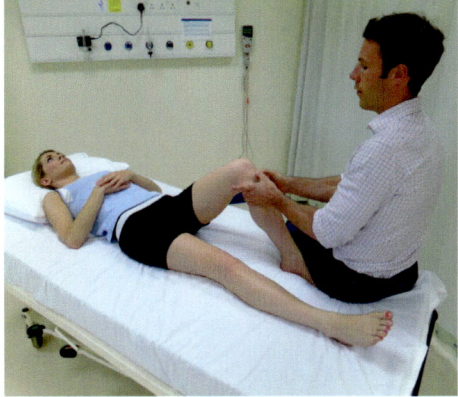

Fig. 16. Anterior drawer test. Pull the tibia forward on the femur to assess ACL integrity.

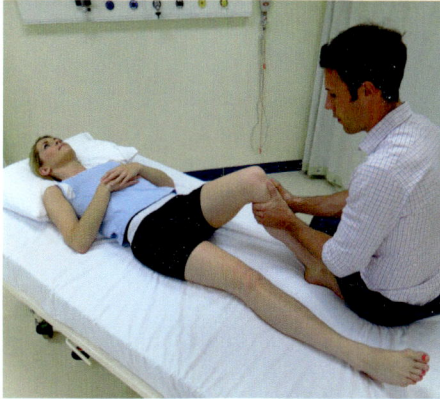

Fig. 17. Posterior drawer test. Push the tibia backwards on the femur to assess PCL integrity.

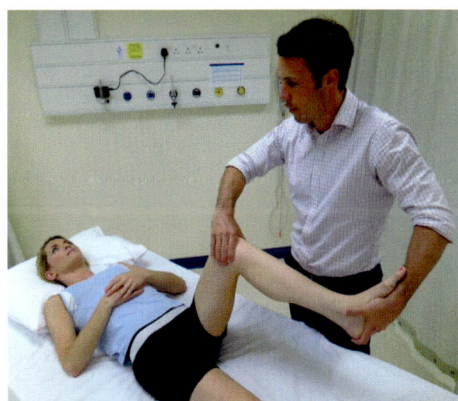

Fig. 18. Collateral ligament stress test. Here the MCL is being assessed for laxity. Swap hands to assess the LCL.

NOTES

17. Ankle & foot notes

Diabetic foot features
- Peripheral neuropathy
  - Particularly loss of ankle jerks & vibration sense on examination
  - Accidental injury & tissue damage
  - Charcot joints (see below)
- Autonomic neuropathy
  - Reduced sweating
  - Dry, cracked skin predisposing to infection
- Arterial insufficiency
  - Large vessel disease
  - Small vessel disease
- All of the above contribute to ulcer formation

Charcot joints
- Also known as neuropathic joints
- Most common cause is diabetic neuropathy
- Other causes:
  - Tabes dorsalis (syphilis – historically a major cause)
  - Cerebral palsy
  - Spinal cord injury
  - Syringomyelia
- Loss of sensation & proprioception to weight-bearing joint results in repeated trauma
- Joint becomes severely damaged & disrupted over time, leading to deformity
- Often still painful despite the neuropathy
- Often associated ulceration and/or infection

Charcot–Marie–Tooth disease
- Group of inherited disorders of the peripheral nervous system
- Mixed motor & sensory peripheral neuropathy
- Progressive loss of muscle tissue & loss of touch sensation
- Foot drop usually present
- Hammer/claw toes
- Muscle wasting in lower legs leads to 'inverted champagne bottle' appearance
- High arched feet (pes cavus) or flat arched feet (pes planus)

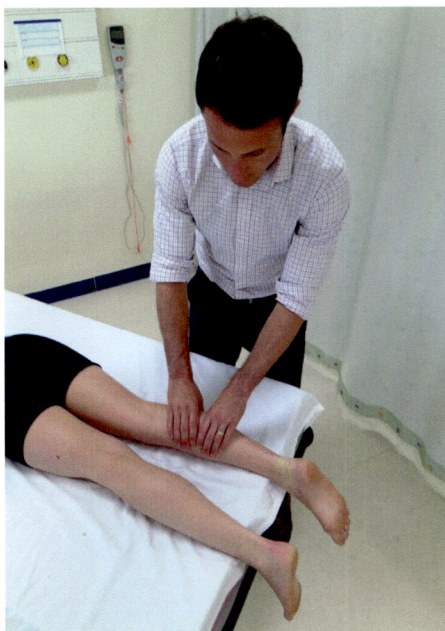

Fig. 19. Simmonds' test. Achilles tendon integrity. Normally you will see foot plantarflexion when you squeeze belly of calf.

NOTES

18. Spine notes
DD Lumbar back pain
NB. Most common in lumbar region
- Non-specific LBP: unknown patho-anatomical cause
- Mechanical
  - Muscular
  - Lumbar sprain or strain
  - Disc herniation
  - OA/arthritic changes/osteophytes
  - # (e.g. osteoporotic wedge #)
  - Spondylolisthesis (vertebral 'slipping')
  - Spinal stenosis
  - Spinal trauma
- Lumbar radiculopathy
  - Radiating front thigh pain: L4 nerve root compression (L1–L3 compression is rare)
  - Radiating posterior buttock/thigh/calf/foot pain/sciatica: L5/S1 nerve root compression/sciatic nerve irritation
- Inflammatory
  - Ankylosing spondylitis
- Other serious pathology
  - Cauda equina syndrome (CES)
  - Bone metastases
  - Myeloma
  - TB
  - Osteomyelitis

Ankylosing spondylitis
- Aetiology
  - Primary
  - Associated with psoriasis/IBD
- 5 males : 1 female (♂ usually severe disease)
- Presents in 20s
- Strong association with HLA-B27
- X-ray findings
  - Sacroiliitis
  - Bamboo spine
- Squaring of vertebrae
- Disc ossification
- Spinal fusion (syndesmophytes)
- Associated features
  - Uveitis
  - Peripheral enthesitis in 33% (especially Achilles tendonitis)
- Management
  - Simple analgesia
  - NSAIDs
  - Anti-TNFα therapy where NSAIDs fail

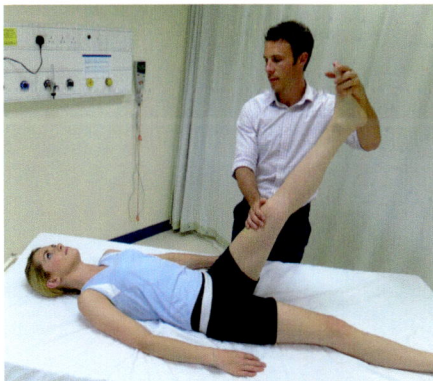

Fig. 20. Straight leg raise. L5/S1 nerve root compression. Watch the patient's face to identify pain.

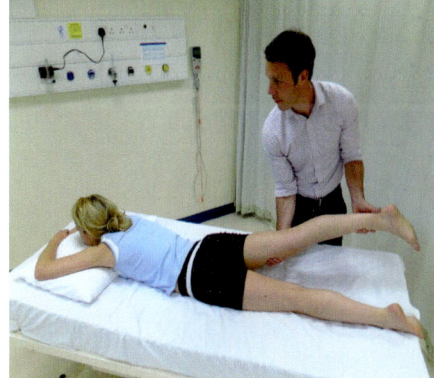

Fig. 21. Femoral stretch test. L4 nerve root compression.

WHY THIS SYSTEM?

Clues/correlations with history	Neuro DDs
• Most neurological-related diagnoses are accompanied by change in functioning, sensation or noticeable strength reduction with either sudden deterioration ± preceding trauma or gradual onset of symptoms	Consider full range of DDs related to acute injury/insult, acute localised or central nerve dysfunction, a chronic or degenerative neurological condition
• One-sided or whole limb weakness/paralysis: face/arm/leg ± speech, persistent or transient	Stroke or TIA
• Head injury ± vomiting/headache/acutely altered mental state	Concussion, TBI, SAH
• Neck or back injury, high-impact fall, acute-onset bilateral muscle weakness/sensory changes below specific spinal cord level ± neck/back pain or risk of malignancy	SCI or lesion, malignancy/metastasis, cord compression or inflammation, e.g. transverse myelitis
• Altered mental state/disorientation/confusion/memory problems ± pain/infection/constipation/decreased oral intake/medication side-effects/change of environment	Delirium, B12/folate deficiency, hypoglycaemia (DM), stroke or TIA, cognitive impairment, dementia
• Headache, neck stiffness, dislike of bright lights, drowsiness ± vomiting, fever, potential seizures or rash	Meningitis, migraine
• LLs: decreased/altered sensation, decreased strength, change in bladder/bowel function, back/LL pain	CES, lumbar stenosis/radiculopathy, vertebral disc herniation, sciatica, LL peripheral neuropathy/nerve injury
• Limb injury with change in limb sensation or function	Peripheral nerve injury related to MSK injury, compartment syndrome
• ULs: decreased/altered sensation, decreased strength, neck/UL pain	Cervical stenosis, vertebral disc herniation, cervical radiculopathy, UL peripheral neuropathy/nerve injury
• Problems with coordinated, refined movement, inc. walking or manual dexterity	Cerebellar ataxia/dysfunction: likely CNS DD; any pathology affecting brain/brainstem can affect cerebellar function dependent on location of affected neurons, e.g. MS, stroke. Toxicity or B12 deficiency [see notes 4b]
• Change in 'normal' function: ability to move about/perform ADLs, maybe unspecific ± obvious weakness	**UMN**, e.g. PD, MS, MND, frontal lobe dementia. **LMN**, e.g. MS, MND, peripheral neuropathy, B12/folate deficiency
• Changed sensation in feet, hands or rising from peripheries ± tripping/unbalanced or reduced dexterity	Peripheral neuropathy (e.g. DM) or demyelinating disease (e.g. MS, GB, CMT)
• Balance problems, dizziness ± nausea, needing to use vision to place limbs accurately	Sensory/proprioceptive loss, vestibular dysfunction, vertigo, UMN lesion, cerebellar dysfunction, MS
• History of toxins/drug history/pharmaceuticals/polypharmacy, e.g. antipsychotics, levodopa	Acute or chronic intoxication, medication-induced side-effects e.g. tremor, dyskinesia, decreased motor function
• Poor diet/self-neglect + change in sensation or function	B12/folate deficiency, malnutrition, dehydration affecting NS function
• Symptoms preceded by period of malaise/virus/infection/fatigue	Viral cause, long Covid, CFS/ME, Lyme disease
• FH of degenerative neurological disease, e.g. Alzheimer's, PD, Huntington's	Alzheimer's, PD, Huntington's
• Repeated episodes of pain, back pain, altered sensations/heightened pain: P+Ns, burning, radiating	Chronic pain condition, vertebral disc herniation, radiculopathy, peripheral neuropathy

! BEFORE starting the examination !

Service user perspective: proactively explore any potential concerns beforehand

- Concern of what will find: explain importance of moving through a series of checks together to help guide what to do next / who to refer to, to move forward with support
- Concern of effort involved / unable to perform certain tests: reassure "do what you can", range of 'expected' in tests correlated with history, not necessarily pathological, one test inconclusive, about looking at the whole picture
- Concern of being tested for physical or mental competence: explain assessment of what possible 'at this time' supported by history (not done to refute it) to gain insight / enable more accurate DDs / more useful action plan
- Concern of pain: check for presence / location of pain, reassure will leave painful area until last. Give explicit permission to ask for examination to be stopped if necessary
- Fear / anxiety about equipment used, e.g. neurotips, tendon hammer: test upfront & explain / reassure
- Concern for exposure: explain the extent of exposure required for tests, reassure about maintaining dignity, offer a chaperone
- Considerations: safety of carrying out specific tests based on history / general inspection, accuracy of findings if in pain, ways to adapt positions to enable safe / effective testing

GENERAL NEUROLOGICAL

GENERAL INSPECTION

Component / action	Examine for	DD / potential findings / extra information
Introduction • Wash / gel hands • Introduce yourself, confirm SU, explain examination • Gain informed consent, explain ability to withdraw, stop the examination, decline specific tests or ask questions • Expose SU to see all 4 limbs sufficiently • Use draping to expose only as required for each examination step		Consider a chaperone or ask "*Would you like to be supported by someone – is there someone in the waiting room?*"
Global inspection As SU arrives / mobilises / rests / transfers: • Look at general movement, balance, posture / positioning, effort Is the movement / posture explained by the history? e.g. congenital disorder / previous stroke, habitual use of walking aids Confirm observations: • "*Do you normally use any walking aids?*" • "*Is this your normal way of walking, do you feel anything has changed?*" • "*Is that how you would normally hold your arm or is that new for you?*"	• Unsteady gait or balance, decreased ability to transfer safely • Obvious weakness / paralysis, holding self up, leaning to one side • Wide stance • Looking at feet when moving or looking where placing limbs • Bradykinesia, flexed extrapyramidal posture, i.e. cannot lie flat (head off pillow), stooped, hands in front • Abnormal effort required, excessive fatigue	→ UMN lesion, stroke, SAH, cerebellar ataxia, degenerative disease (e.g. MS / PD / MND), vestibular dysfunction, sensory / proprioceptive loss, CES. Consider MSK or ENT (inner ear) cause → UMN lesion, stroke, SAH → Cerebellar ataxia, toxicity → Sensory / proprioceptive loss → PD, parkinsonism [see notes 4a] → ME / CFS, long Covid, B12 / folate deficiency, systemic disease / infection. Consider respiratory or cardiovascular cause
Facial expression & speech • Look & listen	• Broken 'staccato' speech or slurring • Poverty of facial expression: 'mask-like', slow monotone speech • Facial drooping or asymmetry	→ Cerebellar dysfunction, toxicity, SAH, stroke, UMN lesion: LMN lesion / bulbar palsy [see Cranial nerves] → PD, parkinsonism [see notes 4a] → Stroke, facial nerve palsy [see Cranial nerves]
Cognitive function • Ability to interact as expected • Consider level of concentration required • State of alertness	• Distracted, difficulty concentrating / following instructions, confusion, fluctuating alertness, paranoia or agitation	→ Head injury / TBI, SAH, stroke, delirium, dementia, meningitis, toxicity, hypoglycaemia (DM), ME / CFS, long Covid, systemic disease or infection. Consider performing CAM [see notes 1]
Involuntary movements • Look	• Muscle fasciculations • Uncontrolled movements • Tremor	→ Brain lesion, UMN or LMN lesion (+ muscle wasting – see below) → Tourette syndrome, movement disorders → PD, parkinsonism, benign tremor, medication-induced, toxicity, anxiety [see notes 2]. Consider GI or respiratory cause, i.e. metabolic flap or flapping tremor

Muscle bulk		
• Inspect & palpate the muscle bulk of all 4 limbs, including palms & back of hands & feet	• Muscle atrophy / wasting	→ LMN / peripheral neuropathy (motor) [see notes 11], myopathy, MND [see notes 3]
		→ CNS: long-standing limb paralysis
• Compare both sides for symmetry: proximal / distal	• Wasting thenar eminence (lateral palm)	→ Carpal tunnel syndrome / median nerve injury
	• Wasting hypothenar eminence (medial palm)	→ Ulnar nerve injury
		→ Consider possible MSK injury / joint disease, deconditioning from disuse
	• Muscle hypertrophy / increased bulk	→ Duchenne muscular dystrophy, e.g. thighs. Steroid use, isometric exercise
Skin inspection		
• Examine hands & feet; peripheral skin & joints	• Soft tissue damage on feet, scald / burn marks on hands	→ Sensory neuropathy [see notes 11]
	• Blisters, ulcers	→ Charcot joints, CMT; consider more detailed examination of ankle & foot [see Musculoskeletal]; consider also vascular cause [see Peripheral vascular]

GENERAL NEUROLOGICAL

CORE EXAMINATION

Component/action	Examine for	DD / potential findings / extra information

Tone
• Support each limb in turn: "*Let your arm/leg go floppy*"
  ○ UL: take SU's hand 'shaking hands' grip, supporting arm at elbow
  ○ LL: hold SU's leg under thigh & around foot
• Move each limb through random, passive ROM to assess resistance
• Aim to move each joint of the limb being tested:
  ○ UL: shoulder, elbow, wrist
  ○ LL: hip, knee, ankle
• Complete for all 4 limbs to ascertain 'normal' for the individual
• Ensure sufficient support of limb & SU in supported position to enhance accuracy of test
	• Hypertonicity: increased resistance or spasticity, clonus (when ankle is suddenly passively dorsiflexed), 'catching', rigidity or jerky ratchet-like movements
	
	• Supinator catch: catching during elbow pronation/supination
	
	• Cogwheel rigidity
	
	• Hypotonicity or flaccidity
		→ UMN pathology: consider individual may struggle to relax, affecting findings
		
		→ Early sign of hypertonicity. UMN lesion
		
		→ PD or parkinsonism: CNS or medication-induced side-effects
		
		→ LMN pathology or acute phase following stroke/brain lesions/SCI, cerebellar lesion (correlate with significant decrease in coordination)

Reflexes
• Using reflex hammer, *rate 0–4+*
• SU must be *relaxed*: can close eyes/look away to facilitate relaxation
 	
ULs (*SU may clench teeth to facilitate upper limb reflex response*)
• **Biceps tendon** (C5,6): forearms supinated on pillow, place fingers centrally over tendon in cubital fossa – tap finger(s) with hammer
• **Triceps tendon** (C6,7): support under upper arm, locate tendon just above olecranon – use hammer directly
• **Brachioradialis tendon** (C5,6): with forearm in mid-prone, place 2 fingers on distal radius, stretch fingers apart – tap most distal finger with hammer or bend wrist & strike directly
 	
LLs (*SU may 'lock fingers & pull' to facilitate lower limb response*)
• **Patellar tendon** (L2,3,4): SU sitting on edge of bed – tap directly with hammer distal to patella
• **Achilles tendon** (S1): hold or place hand under ball of foot, stretch tendon into dorsiflexion – tap directly with hammer at back of ankle
• **Plantar/Babinski test** (L5, S1): use pointed end of hammer to draw line up from heel, along lateral aspect of foot & under toes to hallux
	• NB. 2+ is average response = 'twitch' felt over tendon or subtle movement of limb seen, as described below:
	  ○ Biceps tendon: elbow flexion
	  ○ Triceps tendon: elbow extension
	  ○ Brachioradialis tendon: 'twitch' of tendon > slight hand movement
	  ○ Patellar tendon: knee extension
	  ○ Achilles tendon: tap into hand/plantarflexion
	
	Hyperreflexia
	• 4+ very brisk
	• 3+ brisker than average
	
	Hyporeflexia
	• 1+ diminished
	• 0 absent reflex
	
	• Upward plantar: hallux extension (dorsiflexion) ± toe flaring
		→ Considered 'normal'
		
		→ UMN pathology
		→ May be normal or indicate UMN lesion
		
		→ May be normal or indicate LMN lesion
		→ LMN pathology
		
		→ UMN pathology (not pathological in infant >1–2 years)

GENERAL NEUROLOGICAL

STOP! Think: what do the findings tell you & how much more testing is required?

- What are the positive findings? Correlations?
- Significance of findings in context of history?
- Do history + findings help prioritise DD list?
- Any new DDs/concerns?
- Is neuro referral likely with findings so far?
- Have you localised problem sufficiently, e.g. CNS/PNS or UMN/LMN, affected limb?

[see notes 4, 4a, 4b]

[see notes 5]: Flowchart to aid decision making

GENERAL NEUROLOGICAL

ADDITIONAL EXAMINATION
Choose tests according to priority from a range of options (below) based on clinical reasoning – not necessary to do all

Cues from history/DDs/core examination	Component/action	Examine for	DD/potential findings/extra information
Global functional/movement problems e.g. problem with walking, performing ADLs on feet	**Gait test** • The aim is to look at the parts that make up walking in more detail – which part is a problem? **1. Check 'normal walking' first:** *"Could you walk up & down for me as you normally would?"* • If safe, progress to tests 2–5 below	• Ataxic, wide stance, lacks coordination, instability • Looking at feet • Hemiplegia, foot held in plantarflexion, knee extended, hip abducted to swing through • Shuffling, hesitancy, bradykinesia, loss of arm swing, hurried steps, retropulsion (falling backwards as feet rush ahead) • Insufficient strength to lift LL against gravity • Waddling gait • High/irregular stepping, wide stance, lateral veering • High stepping to clear toes from ground or toes catching on floor • Antalgic gait, limping	→ Cerebellar ataxia, UMN lesion, toxicity → Sensory/proprioceptive dysfunction, peripheral neuropathy [see notes 11] → UMN lesion (stroke, tumour, MS) → PD or parkinsonism → For causes [see notes 9]; also deconditioning, fatigue or systemic illness → Hip muscle weakness (abductors) 2° to peripheral nerve or nerve root lesion (L4–S1), muscular dystrophy → Cerebellar lesion → Foot drop – for causes [see notes 9] → Pain. Consider MSK cause
	2. Heel to toe walking: *"Can you walk as if on a tightrope?"* **3. Walking on heels** **4. Walking on toes** **5. Compare both sides:** a. Single leg stand: *"Can you stand on 1 leg"* b. Single leg knee bend: *"Can you bend the leg you're standing on?"* c. Hop: *"Can you hop?"* *"both sides?"*	• Difficulty or inability to tandem walk • Inability to clear toes off floor or maintain • Inability to go up onto toes or maintain • Inability to perform movement • Equally decreased ability or LL asymmetry	→ Cerebellar dysfunction, UMN lesion, MS, toxicity → Decreased power in dorsiflexors, foot drop: for causes [see notes 9] → Decreased power in plantar flexors/LLs: for causes [see notes 9] → Balance or strength deficit. Consider further testing to narrow down → Bilateral or unilateral LL weakness: for causes [see notes 9] Consider difficult tests to perform if not practised, deconditioning, MSK cause, pain can all affect performance

Balance problems

	Romberg test	• Inability to bring feet together & balance	→ Cerebellar dysfunction / ataxia
	• Standing feet together, eyes closed, hold 20 sec • Protect SU from falling	• Eyes closed: loss of balance / significant sway / sudden loss of balance. Eyes open: balance returns	→ Sensory / proprioceptive loss, vestibular dysfunction (using visual sense to compensate). Consider ENT cause
		• Report of dizziness, nausea	→ Vertigo 2° to brainstem, cerebellar or inner ear dysfunction, BPPV. Consider ENT cause
			Consider systemic disease, fatigue, dehydration, malnutrition, postural hypotension

UMN DD, non-specific or global coordination problems

e.g. problem with walking, performing ADLs on feet	**Pronator drift test**	• In standing: inability to bring feet together & balance	→ Cerebellar dysfunction / ataxia
	• Sitting or standing (feet together), arms outstretched in front with 'palms up', eyes closed, hold 20 sec *"Close your eyes, & keep your arms there"*	• Forearm(s) pronate: ○ Unilateral	→ UMN DD → Motor pathology in brain hemisphere opposite to affected arm
	• Protect SU from unbalancing	○ Bilateral	→ More generalised neurological problem, e.g. bilateral hemispheric or spinal cord damage
	• To challenge, move arms out of position & ask to return to start position	• Sideways or upwards drift of arm(s)	→ Sensory: proprioceptive loss
		• Under- or over-shooting of arm on returning to start position	→ Cerebellar dysfunction
		• Insufficient motor strength to lift limb(s) against gravity or maintain position for 20 sec	→ UMN lesion, neurodegenerative disorder or reduced power from LMN / peripheral nerve dysfunction, deconditioning, fatigue/malaise. Consider MSK, pain

GENERAL NEUROLOGICAL

UL-specific coordination problems / UL limb dysfunction / difficulty with UL-specific tasks / manual dexterity problems			
e.g. doing up buttons, reaching for or grasping an object	**Coordination testing: UL** Perform either or both	• Slow, jerky, non-rhythmic, tremor • Uncoordinated, ataxic • Inconsistent, imprecise • Able to perform with eyes open only	→ PD, parkinsonism, cerebellar dysfunction, benign tremor → Cerebellar dysfunction, UMN lesion or neurodegenerative disorder → LMN lesion / peripheral neuropathy / sensory deficit → Proprioceptive dysfunction
	Point-to-point test: finger–nose • SU touches own nose with index finger, moves from own nose to examiner's stationary finger (SU arm outstretched) • Eyes open, examiner moves finger to challenge SU • Eyes closed to challenge SU, examiner's finger remains in 1 position • Performs several repetitions "*as fast as you can maintain accuracy*"	• Finger–nose: past pointing + tremor as arm stretched out • Finger–nose: insufficient motor strength to lift limb(s) against gravity	→ Cerebellar dysfunction → UMN lesion, neurodegenerative disorder or reduced power from LMN / peripheral nerve dysfunction, deconditioning or fatigue / malaise. Consider MSK, pain
	Rapid alternating movement (RAM) test: hand–thigh • SU moves hand from supination (palm up) to pronation (down) on own thigh • Eyes open, then closed • Performs several repetitions "*as fast as you can maintain accuracy*"	• Hand–thigh: unable to fully supinate	→ UMN DD, neurodegenerative disorder or reduced power: LMN lesion. Consider MSK cause, decreased ROM Consider less dominant side often performs less well (not pathological): Ask "*Are you right- or left-handed?*"

LL-specific coordination problems / LL limb dysfunction or ataxia

e.g. problem with walking, performing ADLs on feet

Coordination testing: LL
Perform either or both

- Slow, jerky, non-rhythmic, tremor → PD, parkinsonism, cerebellar dysfunction, benign tremor
- Uncoordinated, ataxic → Cerebellar dysfunction, UMN lesion or neurodegenerative disorder

- Inconsistent, imprecise → LMN lesion / peripheral neuropathy / sensory deficit
- Able to perform with eyes open only → Proprioceptive dysfunction

Point-to-point test: heel–shin
- SU slides own heel down opposite shin
- Lifts off, brings foot back up onto knee
- Eyes open, then eyes closed to challenge
- Performs several repetitions "*as fast as you can maintain accuracy*"

- Heel–shin: overshooting + tremor → Cerebellar dysfunction

- Heel–shin: insufficient motor strength to lift limb(s) against gravity → UMN lesion or neurodegenerative disorder or reduced power from LMN / peripheral nerve dysfunction, deconditioning or fatigue / malaise. Consider MSK, pain

Rapid alternating movement (RAM) test: foot tap
- SU taps ball of foot on examiner's hand or on floor
- Eyes open, then eyes closed to challenge
- Performs several repetitions "*as fast as you can maintain accuracy*"

- Foot tap: unable to dorsiflex / lift toes to tap, moves at hip not ankle to lift toes → Foot drop [**see notes 9**]

Localised muscle atrophy / limb weakness / decreased limb function (UL / LL / both)

Muscle power testing
Test power relevant to problem, e.g. ULs or LLs based on initial complaint
Can expand testing if required to confirm how widespread problem is

Interpreting findings [see notes 6, 9]
Consider less dominant side often performs less well (not pathological): Ask "*Are you right- or left-handed?*"

- One side of body weakness / limb paralysis → CNS / brain lesion affecting motor cortex / UMN dysfunction, stroke, TIA

- Test according to myotomes [**see notes 7**]
- Compare bilaterally
- Test through ROM against resistance, i.e. not static (isotonic more sensitive than isometric): "*Push me away*", "*pull me towards you*"
- If too weak, test against gravity only
- If SU fails to move, watch / feel for weak muscular contraction
- Grade 0–5 [**see notes 8**]

- UL weakness pattern, inc. shoulder ABduction, elbow / wrist / finger extension → UMN lesion

- All reduced below specific spinal / myotome level → SCI, spinal lesion / compression, or inflammation, e.g. transverse myelitis, Guillain–Barré, CES

- Specific myotomal deficit → Nerve root(s) dysfunction due to spinal DD or problem with surrounding tissues at that level (inflammatory / compressive)
  - Correlate UL with neck complaints, e.g. wrist drop – C7 radiculopathy
  - Correlate LL with back complaints, e.g. foot drop – L5 radiculopathy

GENERAL NEUROLOGICAL

NB. If insufficient time to perform specific power testing, indirect information on power can be gained through making observations in other tests, e.g. gait, pronator drift, coordination tests: is there sufficient power to move against gravity?	• Reduced power/movement in a single limb below a certain joint →	LMN pathology above area of deficit or caused by MSK injury:
		• UL:
		  ○ Weak finger ABduction: ulnar nerve injury at elbow
		  ○ Weak thumb ABduction/opposition: median nerve injury/carpal tunnel
		  ○ Wrist drop or weak wrist extension: radial nerve injury at humerus or 'Saturday night palsy' [see notes 10]
		  ○ Decreased hand/arm/wrist function: brachial plexus injury
		• LL: foot drop [see notes 9]

	• A widespread pattern of reduced power 3/5 or below ± increased fatigue →	UMN lesion or neurodegenerative disorder, malaise from other system cause, chronic pain condition or general deconditioning related to history Consider acute pain as cause of reduced power – not accurate test of muscle power – consider MSK cause

Sensory changes in limbs or peripheral neuropathy DD (UL/LL/both)

e.g.
- reduced or altered sensation
- burning/nagging/shooting/radiating pain

Sensory testing
If no sensory symptoms reported, reason not a priority: examination related to history/DDs
Test sensation relevant to problem, e.g. ULs or LLs based on initial complaint
Can expand testing if required to confirm how widespread problem is

- Ensure SU's eyes closed for tests
- 1st demonstrate sensation on sternum
- Compare bilaterally

Test 1: 'light touch' (use cotton wool)
- Randomly sample L&R dermatomes together [see notes 13]
- "Say YES when you feel me touch your skin"
- "Does it feel the same on both sides?"

Test 1&2

- Reduced on one side/whole limb/large area → CNS pathology/brain lesion affecting sensory cortex, e.g. MS

- Reduced or altered below specific spinal/dermatome level → SCI, spinal lesion/compression, or inflammation, e.g. transverse myelitis, Guillain–Barré, CES

- Reduced or altered in 1 or multiple dermatomes → Nerve root(s) dysfunction due to spinal pathology or problem with surrounding anatomical tissues at that level (inflammatory/compressive)

- Pain or increased sensitivity disproportionate to touch → Acute injury hyperalgesia, pain condition causing chronic hyperalgesia or allodynia (e.g. fibromyalgia), or localised to 1 limb (CRPS), CNS dysfunction (e.g. CPSP)

Interpreting findings [see notes 12]
Peripheral neuropathy [see notes 11]

Test 2: 'sharp/dull' (use neurotip)
- Randomly sample L&R dermatomes together [see notes 13]
- "Say sharp or dull when you feel me touch your skin"
- "Does it feel the same on both sides?"

If suspect peripheral neuropathy perform Test 3

Test 3: distal/proximal across each joint (use cotton wool); start below most distal joint:
- UL: tip of middle finger across DIPJ
- LL: tip of hallux across IPJ
- Work up limb to most proximal joint
- "Tell me if/when you feel the sensation change"
- "Does it feel the same on both sides?"

Temperature (rarely formally assessed)

Test 2:
- Reduced ability to differentiate between sharp ('pain')/dull sensations → Early symptom of peripheral neuropathy: crude (light) touch may be retained though ability to differentiate/sensitivity is reduced. Diabetes, MS

Test 3:
- Reduced or altered sensation in the peripheries → Diabetic neuropathy, peripheral neuropathy [see notes 11], MS

- A distinct sensory level on limb where sensation changes, as move proximally ± tingling, burning, painful sensations below sensory level, often in hands & feet → Local nerve compression or nerve injury related to MSK cause: can test specific distal nerves as part of MSK neurovascular testing [see MSK]

Proprioceptive problems (UL/LL)

e.g. using vision to accurately use UL for tasks or to place feet when moving

Joint position sense testing
Test ULs or LLs relevant to problem
Can expand testing if required to confirm how widespread problem is

- Support SU's hand or foot at both sides with 1 hand
- With other hand, hold distal end of UL or LL at digit:
  - UL: tip of middle finger
  - LL: tip of hallux
- First demonstrate DIP/IP movement: 'up or down' with SU's eyes open
- SU's eyes closed
- Randomly move digit tip up/down 3–4 times & ask SU its position: "Tell me if your finger/toe is up, down or if you're not sure"
- Repeat on other side

- Reduced or inaccurate joint position reporting → Proprioceptive pathway dysfunction as part of sensory NS dysfunction: correlate with findings from other tests to localise to PNS/CNS

GENERAL NEUROLOGICAL

Peripheral sensory changes / peripheral neuropathy DD or sensory changes below specific spinal cord level

e.g. peripheral neuropathy, SCI	**Vibration sense testing**
	Test ULs & LLs bilaterally
	• Strike tuning fork to make it vibrate
	• SU's eyes closed, hold vibrating fork onto:
	  ○ UL: DIP of middle finger
	  ○ LL: IP of hallux
	  ○ Ask "*Can you feel pressure or vibration?*"
	• If pressure > vibration, move proximally up joints of limb until vibration felt:
	  ○ UL: radial styloid → olecranon → shoulder tip
	  ○ LL: medial malleolus → tibial tuberosity → ASIS
		• Inability to sense vibration, or pressure > vibration	→ Peripheral neuropathy, diabetes, SCI
			→ Early symptom of peripheral neuropathy: crude (light) touch may be retained though vibration sense is lost

CNS DDs or recognition problems

	Recognition tests Perform **both** to help localise problem **Stereognosis** (object recognition) • Eyes closed, place an object in SU's hand: "*Can you tell me what that object is?*" **Graphesthesia** (alphanumeric recognition) • Eyes closed, using finger draw a number or letter on SU's palm: "*Can you tell me what number/letter that is?*"	• Inability to recognise & name a 'common' object when placed in hand, with eyes closed • Inability to recognise & name alphanumerics drawn on hand, with eyes closed	→ Dysfunction of sensory cortex → CNS lesion / pathology
Infection or malignancy DD	• Head & neck lymph node examination [see **Appendix: Lymph nodes** for location]	• Lymphadenopathy [see **Appendix: Lymph nodes**]	→ [see **Appendix: Lymph nodes**]

CONCLUSION

Component / action	Examine for	DD / potential findings / extra information
Conclusion • Wash / gel hands • Thank SU, allow them to re-dress, check they are OK • Review observations (HR, BP, RR, SpO$_2$, temperature) • Decide on next steps with the SU or discuss & follow up once reviewed findings		Return to the aim of the examination – to localise the problem by: • Organising & correlating the history & test findings using clinical reasoning • Gathering sufficient information to allow more confident / directed action • Making a final list of DDs / concerns, in order of priority **Action** • Put together a reasoned / safe plan to cover all potential problems identified This could include: 1. Request further tests: e.g. imaging, nerve conduction studies 2. Give advice / take appropriate action within scope 3. Make a referral / consult with MDT 4. Use safeguarding / gain a second opinion where uncertainty 5. Arrange a follow-up

GENERAL NEUROLOGICAL NOTES

1. Confusion assessment method (CAM) – a tool for identifying delirium

A positive or negative result depends on four criteria:
1. **Acute onset and fluctuating course**
   Determined by history taken or repeated assessment
2. **Inattention**
   Reduced ability to maintain attention during backwards count from 20 to 1
3. **Disorganised thinking**
   Disorganised/incoherent speech
4. **Altered level of consciousness**
   From drowsiness to hypervigilance

Positive CAM = 1+2+3 or 1+2+4 or 1+2+3+4

2. DD tremor

- Resting: Parkinsonism
- Flapping: Hepatic failure (encephalopathy), respiratory failure (CO_2 retention), renal failure
- Intention: Cerebellar lesion
- Postural: Benign essential tremor, physiological tremor

3. MND can cause almost any collection of motor signs

Amyotrophic lateral sclerosis (type of MND)
- Weakness ⎫
- Wasting ⎬ LMN signs
- Fasciculation ⎭
- Spasticity ⎫
- Brisk reflexes ⎬ UMN signs

4. Summary of findings: Clinical features of LMN, UMN, extrapyramidal, cerebellar lesion table

	LMN lesion	UMN lesion	Extrapyramidal/parkinsonism	Cerebellar lesion
Tone	Normal or ↓	↑ (spastic)	↑ (rigid)	↓
Reflexes	Reduced	Brisk	Normal	Normal
Plantars	Down	Up	Down	Down
Other features	Wasting Fasciculation	Clonus	Resting tremor Bradykinesia Postural instability	Intention tremor Nystagmus Cerebellar speech
Coordination	Normal	↓	↓	↓↓
Power	↓	↓	Normal	Normal

NOTES

4a. Parkinsonism & related features

Causes of Parkinsonism
- Idiopathic Parkinson's disease
- Drug-induced parkinsonism
  - Lithium
  - Phenothiazine antipsychotics
  - Atypical antipsychotics (less so)
  - Metoclopramide
- Parkinson-plus syndrome
  - Shy–Drager syndrome (autonomic failure)
  - Multi-system atrophy (cerebellar & pyramidal features)
  - Progressive supranuclear palsy (ocular features, including failure of vertical gaze)
- Atherosclerotic pseudoparkinsonism (legs only, less tremor)
- Dementia pugilistica
  - Parkinsonism due to repeated head trauma associated with boxing (e.g. Muhammad Ali)

Core features of parkinsonism (TRAP)
Use this to guide examination sequence:
- **T**remor
- **R**igidity
- **A**kinesia (or more accurately bradykinesia)
- **P**ostural instability

Conditions with similar presentations to parkinsonism
- Benign essential tremor
- Wilson's disease
  - Tremor
  - Dyskinesias
  - Psychiatric illness
  - Hepatotoxicity
  - Kayser–Fleischer rings in eyes

Long-term complications of levodopa therapy
- Increasingly severe parkinsonism
- Autonomic neuropathy
- Dysphagia
- Dementia
- Dyskinesias
- Motor fluctuations (on–off / end of dose)

4b. Cerebellar disease & features

Causes of cerebellar disease
- Stroke
- Tumour
- MS
- Congenital (e.g. Arnold–Chiari)
- Friedreich's ataxia
- Anti-epileptic medication
- Alcohol abuse
- Thiamine deficiency (e.g. Wernicke's encephalopathy)

Classic signs of cerebellar lesion (DANISH)
- **D**ysdiadochokinesis
- **A**taxia (limb / trunk)
- **N**ystagmus
- **I**ntention tremor
- **S**peech (slurred, staccato)
- **H**ypotonia

Wernicke's encephalopathy
- Due to thiamine (vitamin B1) deficiency
- Usually related to alcohol abuse
- If untreated (with IV thiamine replacement) may progress to irreversible Korsakoff's psychosis
- Classical clinical triad
1. Acute confusional state
2. Ophthalmoplegia (especially upgaze)
3. Ataxia (and other cerebellar signs)

Features of cerebellar limb ataxia
- Dysmetria
- Past-pointing
- Intention tremor
- Dysdiadochokinesis

5. Flowchart to aid decision making in neurological examination

Following General inspection and Core examination:
Do you have significant positive findings, e.g. abnormal reflexes, tone and concerns on general inspection correlating with concerns from the history taken?

Yes
↓
Neurological referral is required
↓
Will findings from any further test help strengthen or expedite the referral? [see Additional examination]
Conduct further tests in order to strengthen or expedite referral, e.g. a balance or coordination test finding and/or 1 or 2 further tests to help focus the referral, e.g. power or sensory results that correlate with the initial complaint to help localise the problem
↓
Make an informed referral to neurology

Unsure if significant
↓
Not confident to make a referral
↓
Complete further tests related to the initial complaint [see Additional examination]
e.g. balance or gait testing if a walking or balance problem, coordination or power if problem with specific limb function, sensory testing if altered sensation reported
↓
Specify the deficit, e.g. What movement in the gait test exactly is problematic, is coordination or the power of a limb deficient? Localise the deficit, i.e. which limb and how widespread is the coordination/sensory/power problem? (test selection dependent on initial complaint)
↓
Note all abnormalities found, organise findings and make a referral that demonstrates the main concerns

No
↓
Go back to the history and test the specific deficits reported, e.g. if walking problem reported, test gait to check if any deficits show up under closer inspection, or if sensation a reported problem, test sensation in detail to check for subtle deficits
↓
If no positive findings, consider other systems as the cause, e.g. MSK

6. Guidance on assessing muscle power

Working out the pattern of motor deficit can be difficult and time-consuming. It is essential to correlate with other findings and the history because assessing muscle power is a crude assessment of many elements that make up muscle strength combining:

1. Local musculature: **MSK source**

and

2. **Neuro source:** problem with innervation/message to the muscle:
   - Peripheral nerve (LMN)
   - Nerve roots – myotomes (LMN)
   - Cauda equina (LMN)
   - Spinal cord (UMN)
   - Motor cortex – brain (UMN)

Attempt to localise to CNS or PNS by correlating with other findings.

7. Myotomes

Upper limb		Lower limb	
Nerve root	**Joint action**	**Nerve root**	**Joint action**
C5	Shoulder ABduction	L2	Hip flexion
C5–C6	Elbow flexion	L3	Knee extension
C6	Wrist extension	L4	Ankle dorsiflexion
C7	Elbow extension and/or finger extension	L5	Big toe extension
C8	Finger flexion (gripping)	L5–S1	Hip extension (push heel into bed)
T1	Finger/thumb ABduction	S1	Ankle plantarflexion
		S1–S2	Knee flexion

8. Grading of power (0–5)

5	Normal – full power against resistance
4	Reduced power – able to move against some resistance
3	Able to move against gravity – unable to move against resistance
2	Unable to move against gravity – able to move if gravity eliminated (e.g. can ABduct shoulder when lying supine but not when standing)
1	Visible flicker of muscle contraction, but no movement across joint
0	No muscle contraction

NOTES

GENERAL NEUROLOGICAL NOTES

9. Causes and features of LL motor weakness

DD Unilateral leg weakness
- UMN
  - Stroke
  - Tumour
  - MS
- LMN
  - Root lesion
  - Nerve lesion

DD Foot drop
- LMN lesion or peripheral nerve injury or dysfunction
  - L4/L5 root lesion
  - Sciatic nerve injury (or its branches – peroneal, tibial), e.g. common peroneal nerve injury secondary to MSK cause (proximal fibula # or common peroneal nerve palsy)
  - Peripheral neuropathy
- CES
- Stroke
- MND
- Charcot–Marie–Tooth syndrome

DD Paraparesis = bilateral leg weakness
- Acute & progressive
  - Acute spinal cord compression (UMN)
  - Cauda equina syndrome (LMN)
  - Guillain–Barré syndrome (LMN)
- Spastic paraparesis[1] = bilateral UMN signs
  - Sagittal sinus lesion[2]
    - Parasagittal meningioma
  - Bilateral strokes
  - Syringomyelia (with upper limb signs)
  - Cord trauma
  - Cord compression[3]
    - Extradural tumour
    - Disc prolapse
    - Spondylosis
  - Intrinsic cord disease
    - Tumour
    - Vascular myelopathy
    - MS
- Flaccid paraparesis = bilateral LMN signs
  - Polio
  - Mostly motor peripheral neuropathy
    - Guillain–Barré
    - Lead poisoning
  - Mixed peripheral neuropathy[4] (see below)
    - Charcot–Marie–Tooth
- Mixed UMN & LMN signs = confusing!
  - MND[2]
  - SCDC

[1] Always look for a 'sensory level' on thorax
[2] Exclusively motor signs
[3] Look for LMN signs at level of compression
[4] There will also be marked sensory loss

10. Saturday night palsy

This is the compression of the radial nerve against the humerus caused by falling asleep with your arm over the back of a chair.

11. DD Peripheral neuropathy

- Mostly motor
  - Guillain–Barré
  - Lead poisoning
- Mostly sensory
  - Diabetes mellitus
  - Uraemia (renal failure)
- Mixed (motor/sensory)
  - Charcot–Marie–Tooth
  - B12/folate deficiency (also cause SCDC)
  - Thiamine deficiency
  - Alcohol
  - Vasculitis/SLE
  - Paraneoplastic
  - Amyloid

12. Guidance on assessing sensation

Working out the pattern of sensory deficit can be difficult and time-consuming. It is essential to correlate with other findings and the history because assessing sensation is only a crude assessment of many elements that form functional sensory pathways combining:

- Peripheral nerves (PNS)
- Nerve roots – dermatomes (PNS)
- Cauda equina (PNS)
- Spinal cord (CNS)
- Sensory cortex – brain (CNS)

Attempt to localise to CNS or PNS by correlating with other findings.

NOTES

13. Dermatomes

A note on dermatomes: the exact location of dermatomes will differ slightly in different texts, so when assessing be consistent with one text.

Suggested points for assessing sensation (nerve root dermatomes C4–T1)

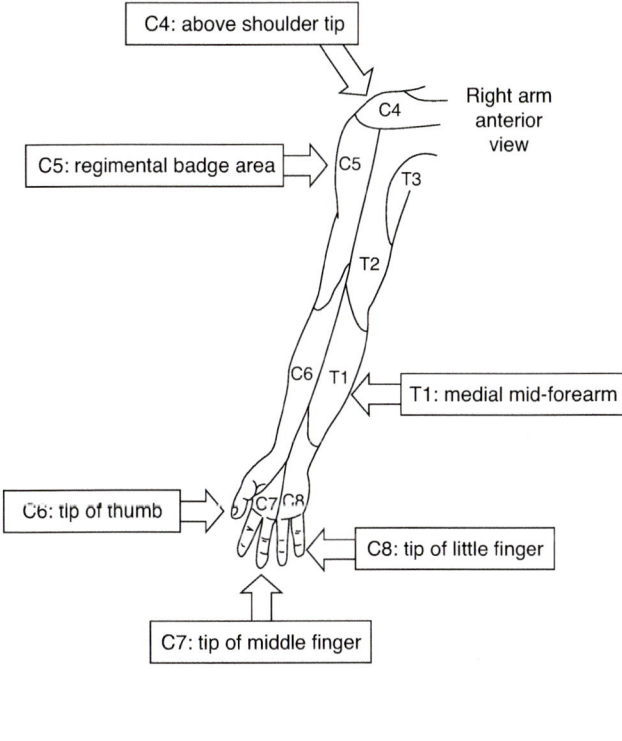

Suggested points for assessing sensation (nerve root dermatomes L2–S1)

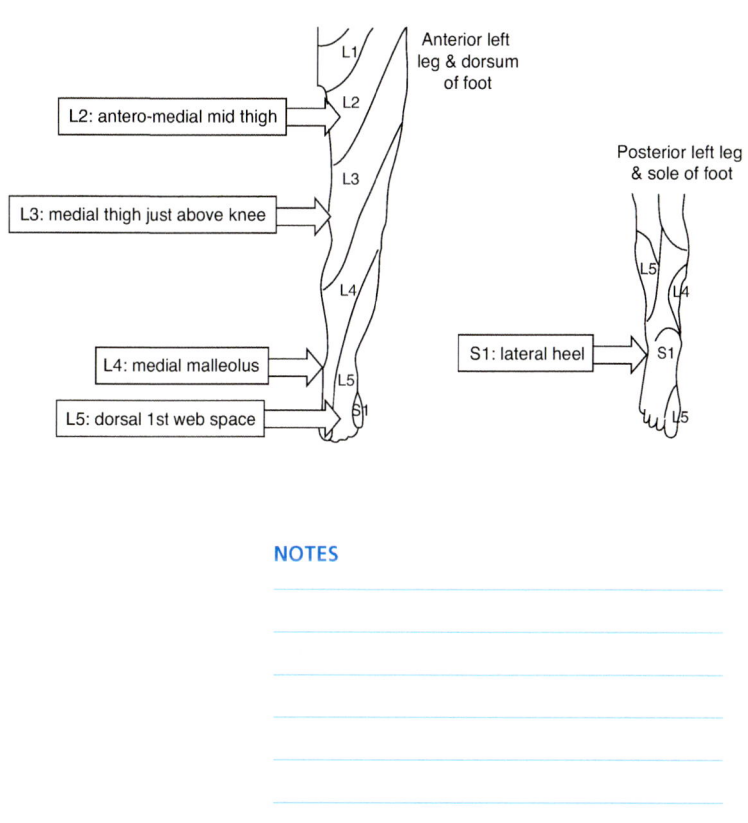

NOTES

CRANIAL NERVES

WHY THIS SYSTEM?

Clues / correlations with history	Cranial nerve DDs
• Isolated deficit relating to specific cranial nerve function, e.g. loss of smell / loss of hearing / eyebrow droop / difficulty turning head	Dysfunction / lesion of the peripheral cranial nerve itself (PNS) 2° to injury / infection / inflammation / tumour or disease, e.g. vasculitis, diabetes, SLE, sarcoidosis, Guillain–Barré syndrome
• Multiple cranial nerve deficits, e.g. change in vision / pupillary reflex / speech / swallow + motor / sensory abnormalities of limbs / problems with or change in function	CNS lesion of brainstem / brain causing cranial nerve dysfunction, e.g. raised ICP, stroke, brain tumour, MS, encephalitis, TBI, SAH, MND NB. Abnormalities in cranial nerve function can help localise the lesion to brain or brainstem; • Olfactory (CN I) & optic (CN II) exit from cerebrum of the brain • Remaining majority (CN III–XII) exit from brainstem
• Change in sense of smell	Olfactory nerve (CN I) lesion or brain lesion, raised ICP, illness-related, e.g. virus / Covid Consider ENT cause [see ENT]
• Change in visual acuity / field / pupillary reflexes	• Optic nerve (CN II) lesion or brain lesion, pituitary adenoma, internal carotid artery aneurysm, GCA, MS, stroke, tumour, abscess • Oculomotor (CN III) nerve lesion or brainstem lesion, raised ICP, PCA aneurysm
• Change in vision / control of eye movements, eye asymmetry	• Oculomotor (III) / trochlear (IV) / abducens (VI) nerve lesion(s) 2° to trauma / diabetes / disease or brainstem lesion, PCA aneurysm, raised ICP • Ophthalmoplegia, ptosis: oculomotor (CN III) nerve palsy, Horner's syndrome, myasthenia gravis
• Generalised visual loss / changes	Optic (CN II) / oculomotor (CN III) / trochlear (CN IV) / abducens (CN VI) nerve dysfunction or palsy, diabetes, hyperglycaemia, ptosis, raised ICP, stroke
• Facial pain, facial / neck rash ± facial weakness / asymmetry • Pain or difficulty eating	Trigeminal neuralgia, trigeminal (CN V) nerve palsy, herpes zoster, Ramsay Hunt syndrome, facial (CN VII) nerve palsy
• Facial drooping or asymmetry	Facial (CN VII) nerve palsy / Bell's palsy, syringobulbia, parotid tumour, sarcoidosis, stroke, TIA
• Change in sense of taste	Facial (CN VII) / glossopharyngeal (CN IX) / vagus (CN X) nerve dysfunction, Ramsay Hunt syndrome, illness-related, e.g. virus; consider ENT cause [see ENT]
• Hearing loss / change or ear pain	Vestibulocochlear (CN VIII) nerve dysfunction, acoustic neuroma, Ramsay Hunt syndrome / herpes zoster oticus [see ENT]
• Difficulty swallowing or eating / chewing	• Bulbar palsy, i.e. LMN lesion to glossopharyngeal (CN IX) / vagus (CN X) / hypoglossal (CN XII) nerve(s) or 2° to, e.g. MND, Guillain–Barré syndrome, syringobulbia, myasthenia gravis, diphtheria, polio • Pseudobulbar palsy / UMN lesion, e.g. stroke, MND, MS, syringobulbia • Facial (CN VII) nerve palsy, trigeminal (CN V) nerve palsy Consider ENT cause [see ENT]

• Difficulty with speech	Dysarthria 2° to: • Bulbar palsy, i.e. LMN lesion to glossopharyngeal (CN IX) / vagus (CN X) / hypoglossal (CN XII) nerve(s) or 2° to, e.g. MND, Guillain–Barré syndrome, syringobulbia, myasthenia gravis • Pseudobulbar palsy / UMN lesion, e.g. stroke, MND, MS, syringobulbia • Facial (CN VII) nerve palsy, trigeminal (CN V) nerve palsy, cerebellar disease, PD
• Difficulty turning head or shrugging shoulders	Spinal accessory (CN XI) nerve lesion 2° to trauma, infection, tumour, iatrogenic injury, e.g. radiation therapy, surgical procedures or Guillain–Barré syndrome Possible MSK cause [see MSK] (cervical spine / shoulder)
• History of head injury / trauma or possible head trauma	SAH, TBI, raised ICP, concussion

! BEFORE starting the examination !

SU perspective: proactively explore any potential concerns beforehand

- Concern of what will find: explain importance of moving through a series of tests to gain insight & make a more useful action plan: what to do next / who to refer to
- Concern of ability to perform certain tests: reassure "*do what you can*", range of 'expected' in tests correlated with history given
- Concern of pain: check for presence / location of pain, reassure; give explicit permission to ask for examination to be stopped if necessary
- Fear / anxiety about equipment used, e.g. neurotips – test upfront & explain / reassure

CRANIAL NERVES

GENERAL INSPECTION

Component / action	Examine for	DD / potential findings / extra information
Introduction • Wash / gel hands • Introduce yourself, confirm SU, explain examination • Gain informed consent, explain ability to withdraw, stop the examination, decline specific tests or ask questions • Expose SU to shoulders; use draping to expose only as required for each examination step		Consider a chaperone or ask *"Would you like to be supported by someone – is there someone in the waiting room?"*
Global inspection • As SU arrives / moves around: • Ask *"Has your vision changed recently?"* • Ask *"Has your hearing changed recently?"*	• Difficulty with vision – squinting • Difficulty navigating way, using hands for guidance, bumping into things • Lifting head to see where going or overcompensating with bodily movements to gain visual accuracy • Turning body rather than head to see things • Difficulty with hearing • Difficulty with balance	→ Cranial nerve palsy II, III, IV, VI (IV & VI single palsies rare) → Change in vision due to cranial nerve palsy II, III, IV, VI; consider central cause [see **General neurological**] → Ptosis: oculomotor (CN III) nerve palsy, ophthalmoplegia [see **notes 2**] → Possible spinal accessory (CN XI) nerve lesion, likely MSK cause → Vestibulocochlear (CN VIII) nerve dysfunction [go to **ENT**] → Consider inner ear related cause [see **ENT**]; consider central cause, e.g. stroke, MS, cerebellar lesion [see **General neurological**]
Cognitive function • State of alertness / ability to interact as expected	• Inattention, difficulty following instructions, confusion, fluctuating alertness / drowsiness	→ Stroke, concussion, TBI, SAH, raised ICP
Look ± palpate • Around circumference of skull **Look** • Face, neck, shoulders	• Signs of head injury: swelling / lacerations / bleeding / deformity • Localised facial or neck trauma / scarring or inflammation • Rash • Any obvious facial weakness or asymmetry	→ Risk of potential CNS lesion ± cranial nerve deficit 2° to injury; consider additional neurological examination [see **General neurological**] → Acute trauma, prior surgery or infection correlating with peripheral cranial nerve(s) injury → Herpes zoster / Ramsay Hunt syndrome → Facial (CN VII) nerve palsy / Bell's palsy, Ramsay Hunt syndrome; consider UMN lesion: stroke, TIA [see **General neurological**]

A note on cranial nerve examination

Cranial nerve examination can be carried out in full or in part based on the history and/or deficit reported.

- Generally, a singular cranial nerve deficit indicates a peripheral nerve lesion & may warrant only partial examination guided by the cranial nerve groups below.
- Multiple cranial nerve deficits, plus motor/sensory abnormalities of limbs/problems with or change in function, may indicate a central brain/brainstem lesion indicating full examination + further neurological examination [**see General neurological**].
- A history of head injury or possible head trauma where there is a risk of a CNS lesion, indicates more extensive cranial nerve examination + potential further examination [**see General neurological**].

CORE EXAMINATION – SELECT ACCORDING TO DDS/HISTORY

Component/action	Examine for	DD / potential findings/extra information
Sense of smell: CN I olfactory nerve		
• Ask "*Have you noticed any changes in your sense of smell?*"	• Report of reduced sense of smell	→ Olfactory nerve palsy 2° to local cause, e.g. nasal polyps, tumour, prior surgery or central cause, e.g. frontal lobe tumour, meningitis
• Inspect briefly the forehead, nose & surrounding area	• Trauma/inflammation/nasal discharge	→ Olfactory nerve palsy 2° to trauma or infection (URTI most common) [**see ENT**]
Visual function: CN II optic, CN III oculomotor, CN IV trochlear, CN VI abducens		
Ask:		
• "*Do you wear glasses or contact lenses?*" – ensure glasses on/contact lenses in if normally worn, to assess 'normal' visual ability	• Report of reduced/change in vision	→ Change in vision due to cranial nerve palsy II, III, IV, VI; consider central cause, e.g. stroke, MS [**see General neurological**]
• "*Have you had any problems with your vision recently?*"	• Trauma, inflammation	→ Acute injury, infection, orbit trauma – possible trochlear (CN IV) nerve damage
Inspect:	• Asymmetrical eyebrows or expression	→ Bell's palsy, LMN facial (CN VII) nerve lesion (see Facial function exam below)
• Around the eyes		
• Eyebrows	• Unilateral ptosis (upper eyelid droop)	→ Oculomotor (CN III) nerve palsy (complete or partial), congenital, diabetic oculomotor (CN III) nerve palsy, Horner's syndrome [**see notes 3**]
• Eyelids	• Bilateral ptosis (upper eyelid droop)	→ External ophthalmoplegia [**see notes 2**], myasthenia gravis, myotonic dystrophy, congenital
• Gaze	• Strabismus/asymmetrical gaze or deviated 'down & out'	→ Oculomotor (CN III) nerve palsy (complete or partial), Horner's syndrome, congenital
• Pupils	• Dilated pupil (fixed), asymmetrical pupils	→ Complete oculomotor (CN III) nerve palsy 2° to, e.g. PCA aneurysm, raised ICP with tentorial herniation
	• Unilateral miosis (constricted pupil) + ptosis	→ Horner's syndrome [**see notes 3**]
	• Bilateral miosis (constricted pupils)	→ Opioid/barbiturate consumption
• Sclera, cornea, iris, conjunctiva – for colour & moisture	• Redness of the sclera	→ Dryness, irritation, uveitis
	• Pale conjunctiva or discoloured sclera (yellowing)	→ Consider systemic disease [**see GI/Respiratory**]

CRANIAL NERVES

Test:
- Visual acuity (CN II)
  - Use Snellen chart (ideally) or other reading material
  - Advise *"Hold this at relaxed arm's length distance away"* (NB. This is a crude test of visual acuity – you would usually use a Snellen chart at 6m distance away)
  - Ask *"Which is the lowest line you are able to read with…"*
    1. Both eyes
    2. Left eye *"Cover your right eye with your right hand"*
    3. Right eye *"Cover your left eye with your left hand"*
    Ask *"Has this changed from your normal vision?"*

  - Report of change in 'normal' or difficulty with reading using visual aids / inability to read 6/12 or 20/40 line on the Snellen chart with visual aids (UK driving test standard) → Optic (CN II) nerve palsy 2° to optic neuritis, MS, GCA, glaucoma, macular degeneration, diabetic retinopathy or central cause, e.g. stroke, MS; refer for more accurate eye testing
  - Loss of vision in 1 eye → Optic (CN II) nerve palsy causing monocular blindness 2° to optic neuritis, MS, GCA, glaucoma, macular degeneration, diabetic retinopathy, stroke

- Peripheral vision / visual fields in 4 quadrants (CN II)
  - Advise *"Look at my nose & keep looking there"*
  - Instruct *"When you see my fingers appear in your peripheral vision, indicate with your own finger on that side or both sides"*
  - Starting with hands to side of SU's head, wiggle both index fingers, slowly bringing them in bilaterally toward SU's visual field from:
    1. Above SU's head
    2. At SU's ear level
    3. Below SU's chin

  - Inattention – only seeing one finger move → Stroke, concussion, TBI, SAH, raised ICP
  - 'Tunnel vision' or outer visual field loss bilaterally → Optic (CN II) nerve palsy causing bitemporal hemianopia 2° to, e.g. pituitary adenoma, internal carotid artery aneurysm, acute head injury
  - Visual field loss on the same side bilaterally, e.g. left or right on both sides → Optic (CN II) nerve palsy causing homonymous hemianopia 2° to anything behind optic chiasm (where optic nerves cross) or stroke, tumour, abscess, acute head injury, demyelinating disease, e.g. MS

- Pupillary light reflex – direct and consensual (CN II, III)
  - Advise *"I am going to briefly shine my torch into your eyes – place a flat hand over your nose to separate your eyes"*
  - First check pupil size
  - Shine pen light over one eye & check pupil reaction
  - Same eye (direct) & other eye (consensual)
  - Repeat for both eyes
  - Swinging torch test: repeatedly move torch between eyes

  - Pupil(s) remains dilated & unresponsive to light → Complete oculomotor (CN III) nerve palsy / optic nerve palsy 2° to, e.g. PCA aneurysm, raised ICP with tentorial herniation
  - Pupil spared & reacts appropriately → Diabetic oculomotor (III) nerve palsy
  - Diminished or no pupil constriction followed by inappropriate dilation in one or both eyes → Relative afferent pupil defect (RAPD) / Marcus Gunn pupil (MGP) 2° to, e.g. optic (CN II) nerve palsy, optic neuropathy, retinal disease, MS, glaucoma, stroke

- Eye movements (CN III, IV, VI)
  - Advise "*Keep your head still & follow my finger with your eyes*"
  - Slowly move a pen in an H-pattern in front of SU (approx. arm's length from face) – first go slowly!

  - Then move quickly to elicit nystagmus

- Difficulty with gaze to end of range ± diminished eye coordination → Ophthalmoplegia [**see notes 2**]
- Difficulty with vertical up/down gaze → Progressive supranuclear palsy
- Unable to look upward – failure of upward gaze → Wernicke's encephalopathy
- Both eyes not coordinating when looking to the side (uncoordinated lateral gaze) → Internuclear ophthalmoplegia [**see notes 2**]
- Nystagmus/involuntary eye movement → Brainstem lesion, e.g. MS, stroke, tumour, internuclear ophthalmoplegia [**see notes 2**] or cerebellar disease [**see General neurological**]
  - → Vestibular apparatus problem, e.g. labyrinthitis, Ménière's disease, CN VIII lesion [**see ENT**]
  - → Can be congenital (tends to cause rhythmical pendular nystagmus most marked in neutral position)
  - → NB. Slight nystagmus may occur at extremes of 'normal' lateral gaze

  - "*Tell me if you see double at any point*"
  - If seeing double ask if images are:
    - separated horizontally or vertically
    - still visible, if you cover each eye in turn

- Diplopia → Oculomotor (CN III), trochlear (CN IV), abducens (CN VI) nerve palsy, diabetic oculomotor (CN III) nerve palsy, ophthalmoplegia [**see notes 2**]
  - → Note any specifics of diplopia for referral to ophthalmology

- Accommodation (CN III, IV, VI)
  - "*Keep looking at my finger as I move it towards you*"
  - Start approx. arm's length from SU's face, move finger slowly in towards SU's nose
  - Check that pupils constrict appropriately

- Diminished or absent pupil constriction as finger moves towards SU – convergence insufficiency → Age-related changes, eye strain, underlying risk factors: diabetes, MS. NB. Convergence is preserved in internuclear ophthalmoplegia [**see notes 2**]

CRANIAL NERVES

Facial function: CN V trigeminal, CN VI facial

Inspect: face: muscle bulk	• Muscle wasting, asymmetrical bulk, hollowed effect	→ Chronic nerve palsy: trigeminal (CN V) / facial (CN VII) 2° to LMN or UMN lesion
Trigeminal (CN V) Inspect: face & around ears	• Visible discomfort, holding face / jaw, tentative to move jaw or be touched on face • Facial rash • Rash in/around 1 ear ± facial weakness on same side / hearing loss	→ Trigeminal neuralgia, herpes zoster, Ramsay Hunt syndrome; consider TMJ disorder or acute injury / # / dislocation → Herpes zoster → Ramsay Hunt syndrome / herpes zoster oticus

Test sensation:
• Ensure SU's eyes closed for tests
• 1st demonstrate sensation on hand
• Compare bilaterally in ophthalmic, maxillary & mandibular zones [**see notes 4**]
  1. Test '**light touch**' (use cotton wool)
     "Say YES when you feel me touch your face" – "Does it feel the same on both sides?"
  2. Test '**sharp / dull**' (use neurotip)
     "Say SHARP or DULL when you feel me touch your face" – "Does it feel the same on both sides?"
	• Reduced / altered sensation or ability to differentiate between sharp ('pain') / dull sensations
	
	• Pain or increased sensitivity disproportionate to touch
		→ Trigeminal (CN V) nerve palsy 2° to trigeminal neuralgia, herpes zoster, acoustic neuroma, nerve compression: local tumour / cyst, nerve trauma (injury, ENT surgery), demyelinating disease, e.g. MS
		→ Trigeminal neuralgia, herpes zoster, local nerve injury / compression, TMJ disorder or acute trauma

Test motor function:
• Ask "*Open your mouth against my hand*" – gently push upwards on bottom of SU's chin
 	
• Ask "*Move your jaw side to side*" – with hands each side of jaw, gently resist this movement
• Ask "*Clench your jaw*" – palpate temporalis & masseter muscles [**see notes 5**]
• Reflex: jaw jerk
  ○ Ask: "*Let your mouth hang open*"
  ○ Place your thumb on SU's chin – "*I'm going to tap your chin, keep your mouth open & relaxed*"
  ○ Strike thumb briskly with tendon hammer
	• Reduced strength / asymmetry – jaw will deviate towards side of weakness
	
	• Pain or hesitancy to move jaw
	
	• Muscle wasting, asymmetrical bulk
	
	• Brisk = abnormal reflex (minimal / absent = normal)
		→ LMN trigeminal (CN V) nerve lesion / palsy 2° to trigeminal neuralgia, herpes zoster, acoustic neuroma, nerve compression – local tumour / cyst, nerve trauma (injury, ENT surgery), demyelinating disease, e.g. MS
		
		→ Trigeminal neuralgia, TMJ disorder or acute trauma
		→ Trigeminal (V) nerve palsy 2° to longer-term cause e.g. demyelinating disease or chronic pain disorder (TMJ, trigeminal neuralgia)
		→ UMN lesion, e.g. stroke / tumour / MS, etc. [**see General neurological**]
		Assess bulbar function – correlate with findings for pseudobulbar palsy / UMN lesion [**see notes 6**]

Facial (CN VII)
Inspect: facial tone

- Asymmetry / drooping with loss of forehead & eyebrow → Bell's palsy – LMN facial (CN VII) nerve lesion 2° to, e.g. movements / reduced forehead wrinkling ± eyelid parotid tumour, herpes zoster, Ramsay Hunt syndrome, droop / inability to close eye sarcoidosis (often bilateral), syringobulbia
- Asymmetry / drooping with forehead spared → UMN lesion, e.g. stroke, TIA, brain tumour, syringobulbia impacting on brainstem [see **General neurological**]
- Drooping of corner of mouth / loss of nasolabial fold → LMN or UMN lesion causing facial (CN VII) nerve palsy (smile lines)

Test sensory function:
- Ask "*Have you noticed any change in taste recently?*" • Report of change in taste → Facial (CN VII), glossopharyngeal (CN IX) / vagus (CN X) nerve dysfunction, Ramsay Hunt syndrome, illness-related, e.g. virus; consider ENT cause [see **ENT**]
- Ask "*Are you troubled by loud noises? – Is this new?*" • Report of new sensitivity to loud noises → Facial (CN VII) nerve dysfunction, tinnitus [see **ENT**]

Test motor function:
- Observe facial expressions • Reduced ability to perform facial expressions → LMN or UMN lesion causing facial (CN VII) nerve palsy
  - "*Raise your eyebrows*", "*Screw up your eyes*"
  - "*Frown, smile, show your teeth*"
- Ask "*Close your eyes tightly*" – "*Don't let me open* • Unable to keep eyes closed – Bell's sign: upgaze on → Bell's palsy – LMN facial (CN VII) nerve lesion *them*" attempted eye closure
- Ask "*Puff out cheeks*" – palpate for firmness / symmetry • Unable to puff out 1 side / asymmetry → LMN or UMN lesion causing facial (CN VII) nerve palsy

CRANIAL NERVES

Bulbar function: CN IX glossopharyngeal, CN X vagus, CN XII hypoglossal

Assessment	Finding	Interpretation
Ask "*Have you noticed any change in taste recently?*"	Report of change in taste	Glossopharyngeal (CN IX) / vagus (CN X) / facial (CN VII) nerve dysfunction, Ramsay Hunt syndrome, illness-related, e.g. virus; consider ENT cause [see ENT]
Inspect:		
• Outside of mouth	Drooling, trembling / twitching lips	Bulbar (LMN lesion) or pseudobulbar (UMN lesion) palsy [see notes 6]
• Inside mouth using pen torch	Inflammation / ulceration	Infection [see ENT]
• Tongue appearance	Flaccid, wasted & fasciculating tongue	Bulbar palsy, i.e. LMN lesion to glossopharyngeal (CN IX) / vagus (CN X) / hypoglossal (CN XII) nerve(s) or 2° to MND, myasthenia gravis, Guillain–Barré syndrome, diphtheria, polio, syringobulbia
	Spastic, contracted slow-moving tongue	Pseudobulbar palsy / UMN lesion, e.g. MND, stroke, MS, syringobulbia impacting on brainstem [see General neurological]
Check		
• Soft palate movement: "Say '*ahhh*'" & look at movement of uvula	Uvula deviation – pulls away from side of weakness	Vagus (CN X) nerve lesion. NB. can be normal or infectious cause [see ENT]
• Tongue movements: "*Stick your tongue straight out*" "*Move your tongue from side to side*"	Tongue deviation or difficulty moving to 1 side	Hypoglossal (CN XII) / vagus (CN X) nerve palsy – deviates towards side of weakness
• Swallow: Ask SU to swallow a sip of water	Choking, coughing, or difficulty swallowing	Dysphagia or aspiration 2° to bulbar or pseudobulbar deficit; consider inflammatory or structural occlusion [see ENT]
Speech (assessed throughout)		
• Ask "*Has your speech or voice changed?*"	Dysarthria	Bulbar or pseudobulbar palsy, facial (CN VII) nerve palsy (correlate with facial weakness), myasthenia gravis, cerebellar dysfunction, PD [see General neurological]
	Dysphonia	Bulbar or pseudobulbar palsy; consider ENT cause

Neck & shoulder function: CN XI spinal accessory

Assessment	Finding	Interpretation
Inspect: neck & shoulders – muscle bulk	Muscle wasting, dropped shoulder – asymmetrical	Chronic spinal accessory (CN XI) nerve palsy 2° to LMN lesion or prior stroke / injury
Test motor function:	Muscle wasting, dropped shoulder(s) – symmetrical	Progressive disease, e.g. MND, MS, sarcopenia (frailty)
• Trapezius: "*Lift both your shoulders up towards your ears (shrug your shoulders)*" Resist the movement on both sides at the same time	Reduced strength or ROM / asymmetry	Spinal accessory (CN XI) nerve palsy 2° to trauma / injury, infection, tumour, iatrogenic injury, e.g. radiation therapy, surgical procedures (lymph node biopsy, central line insertion, neck dissection surgery)
• Sternocleidomastoid: "*Turn your head to look over your shoulder*" Gently resist the movement by placing hand against SU's chin Repeat on both sides		Guillain–Barré syndrome, MND, MS [see General neurological]
		Consider MSK cause: neck / shoulder [see MSK]

Hearing: CN VIII vestibulocochlear

[see ENT]

ADDITIONAL EXAMINATION

Choose tests according to priority from a range of options (below) based on clinical reasoning – not necessary to do all

Cues from history/DDs/core examination	Component/action	Examine for	DD / potential findings/extra information
Positive findings from examination of trigeminal (CN V) or facial (CN VII) nerve(s) or DD of brainstem lesion	**Corneal reflex test (blink reflex)** Either • **Direct** ○ Ask SU to remove contact lenses/glasses ○ Ask SU to "*look up*" whilst you gently depress the lower eyelid ○ Lightly touch the edge of the cornea (not the conjunctiva) using a wisp of damp cotton wool ○ Look for both direct & consensual blinking OR • **Indirect** ○ Can be done if 'Direct' is deemed too intrusive ○ Test nostril sensation by sweeping a wisp of cotton wool inside the base of the nostril (repeat in both nostrils)	• Absent or abnormal reflex, i.e. does not elicit blinking in eye touched or in both eyes ○ Same eye as side of trigeminal or facial nerve symptoms ○ Bilateral • Absent or abnormal blink reflex, i.e. does not elicit both direct & consensual blinking ○ Same eye as side of trigeminal nerve symptoms ○ Bilateral	→ LMN trigeminal (CN V) or facial (CN VII) nerve(s) lesion, e.g. glaucoma, diabetes (peripheral neuropathy); correlate with findings from Facial function testing → UMN lesion, e.g. brainstem [**see General neurological**] → LMN trigeminal (CN V) nerve lesion; correlate with findings from trigeminal (CN V) nerve testing → UMN lesion, e.g. brainstem [**see General neurological**]
Infection or malignancy DD	**Head & neck lymph node examination** [**see Appendix: Lymph nodes** for location]	Lymphadenopathy [**see Appendix: Lymph nodes**]	→ [**see Appendix: Lymph nodes**]

CRANIAL NERVES

CONCLUSION

Component / action	Examine for	DD / potential findings / extra information
Conclusion • Wash / gel hands • Thank SU, allow them to re-dress, check they are OK • Review observations (HR, BP, RR, SpO$_2$, temperature) • Decide on next steps with the SU or discuss & follow up once reviewed findings		Return to the aim of the examination – to localise the problem by: • Organising & correlating the history & test findings using clinical reasoning • Gathering sufficient information to allow more confident / directed action • Making a final list of DDs / concerns, in order of priority Action • Put together a reasoned / safe plan to cover all potential problems identified This could include: 1. Request further tests, e.g. imaging – CT head 2. Give advice / take appropriate action within scope 3. Make a referral / consult with MDT 4. Use safeguarding / gain a second opinion where uncertainty 5. Arrange a follow-up

1. Causes of grouped cranial nerve palsies

- Cerebellopontine angle tumour (acoustic neuroma or meningioma)
  - Corneal reflex lost first (CN V)
  - Then CN VII & VIII
  - Then rest of CN V
  - Sometimes CN IX & X
- Paget's disease of bone (bony impingement on nerves)
  - CN V, VII & VIII
- Gradenigo's syndrome (complication of otitis media)
  - CN V & VI
- Syringobulbia
  - Bulbar palsy (CN IX, X & XII)
  - CN VIII – vertigo & nystagmus
  - CN V – facial pain/sensory loss
  - CN VII sparing
  - May have Horner's syndrome
  - May have syringomyelia
- Cavernous sinus thrombosis
  - CN III, IV & VI (VI most common)
  - CN V – pain (especially ophthalmic division)
  - Corneal reflex may be lost (CN V)
  - Also headache, periorbital oedema, proptosis

NOTES

2. Ophthalmoplegia

DD Ophthalmoplegia
i.e. **paralysis / weakness of the eye muscles** caused by:
- Cranial nerve palsy – oculomotor (CN III), trochlear (CN IV), abducens (CN VI)

Specific causes:

- ↑ICP

- Myasthenia gravis

- Graves' disease (autoimmune cause of hyperthyroidism)

- Progressive supranuclear palsy – characterised by difficulty with vertical (up / down) gaze [see **General neurological notes 4a**]

- Wernicke's encephalopathy – characterised by failure of upward gaze [see **General neurological notes 4a**]

DD External (extranuclear) ophthalmoplegia
Commonly a result of chronic disease causing peripheral cranial nerve palsy, e.g.
- Mitochondrial disease
- Myopathy

Presentation:
- Typically bilateral, symmetrical ptosis, pupil spared
- Difficulty controlling eye coordination
- Incidence age 18–40 years
- Slow progression over time = chronic / progressive external ophthalmoplegia (C/PEO)
- May be accompanied by generalised muscle weakness / decreased exercise tolerance (myopathy of neck, arms, legs), dysphagia

DD Internuclear ophthalmoplegia (INO)
Cranial nerve palsy resulting from a central cause, e.g.
- Brainstem lesion
- ↑ICP
- MS (almost always the cause in a young SU)
- Stroke
- Lyme disease (rare)
- Tricyclic antidepressant overdose (rare)

Features:
- Disorder of coordinated lateral gaze
- Causes failure of ADduction of eye on affected side
- In a left-sided INO:
  - Lateral gaze to left is normal (left eye is being ABducted)
  - On attempting to look to the right:
    - Right eye ABducts normally
    - Left eye fails to ADduct and remains looking straight ahead
    - Right eye consequently displays nystagmus as it attempts to compensate
- Convergence is preserved (i.e. the left eye can ADduct normally as long as the goal is not lateral gaze)

3. DD Horner's syndrome
- Central lesion
  - Stroke/tumour/MS
  - Syringobulbia
- T1 root lesion
  - Spondylosis
  - Neurofibroma
- Brachial plexus lesion
  - Pancoast tumour
  - Cervical rib
  - Trauma/birth injury (Klumpke's)
- Neck lesion
  - Tumour
  - Carotid artery aneurysm
  - Sympathectomy
- With cluster headaches

4. Branches of the trigeminal nerve to test sensation

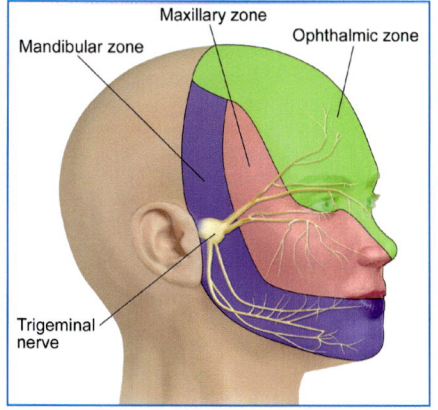

Reproduced from www.geekymedics.com under a CC-BY-SA licence (BruceBlaus).

5. Temporalis & masseter muscles

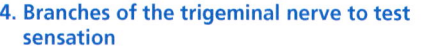

NOTES

6. Features of bulbar & pseudobulbar palsies

NB. Bulbar palsy refers to a range of symptoms linked to impairment of the glossopharyngeal (CN IX), vagus (CN X), accessory (CN XI), and hypoglossal (CN XII) cranial nerves, which control muscles involved in swallowing, speech & facial movements

	Lesion Use to correlate with other LMN/UMN findings from general neurological examination	**Aetiology** ** NB. MND, syringobulbia can present with both LMN & UMN findings	**Tongue appearance** (use to differentiate)	**Other features**
Bulbar palsy	LMN	• MND** • Syringobulbia** • Diphtheria • Polio • Myasthenia gravis • Guillain–Barré syndrome	• Flaccid • Wasted • Fasciculating	• Drooling • Dysarthria • Dysphagia • Dysphonia • Tremulous lips
Pseudobulbar palsy	UMN	• MND** • Syringobulbia** • Bilateral strokes (e.g. internal capsule) • MS	• Spastic • Contracted • Slow-moving	• Drooling • Dysarthria • Dysphagia • Dysphonia • Emotional lability

NOTES

PERIPHERAL VASCULAR

WHY THIS SYSTEM?

Clues/correlations with history	Peripheral vascular DDs
• Pain in the arms or legs	Peripheral arterial disease (PAD)
• Cramping pain in arms or legs with activity	Intermittent claudication
• Cold, numbness, pallor in the arms or legs	PAD
• Colour change in fingers or toes in cold weather	Raynaud's disease
• Skin changes (eczema, thinning)	Venous insufficiency (VI) or PAD [see notes 1]
• Swelling in calves, legs or feet	VI, DVT
• Slow-healing wounds on lower legs	Venous or arterial ulceration [see notes 1]
• Older age, high BMI, FH of VI, female gender, reduced mobility, PMH of DVT	Increased risk of VI
• Older age, hypertension, diabetes, high BMI, FH of PAD, hyperlipidaemia, smoking history	Increased risk of PAD

! BEFORE starting the examination !

SU perspective: proactively explore any potential concerns beforehand

- Concern for exposure: explain the extent of exposure required, reassure about maintaining dignity, offer a chaperone
- Concern about appearance of/condition of wounds on lower limbs: acknowledge and reassure around the need for assessment to make an informed shared decision
- Anxiety about serious findings, e.g. DVT, ischaemia that threatens viability of limb: explain the importance of moving through a series of checks together to help guide what to do next/who to refer to in order to move forward with support
- Minimise position changes if older adult

GENERAL INSPECTION

Component/action	Examine for	DD/potential findings/extra information
Introduction • Wash/gel hands • Introduce yourself, confirm SU, explain examination • Gain informed consent, explain ability to withdraw, stop the examination, decline specific tests or ask questions • Use draping to expose only as required for each examination step		Consider a chaperone or ask "*Would you like to be supported by someone – is there someone in the waiting room?*"
General appearance	• Unwell/distressed/in pain • Missing limbs, digits, prosthesis • Dressings, scars	→ Amputation secondary to critical ischaemia → Healing/healed ulcers
Hands	• Peripheral cyanosis • Tendon xanthomata	→ Poor perfusion → Hypercholesterolaemia
Nails	• Nailfold infarcts	→ Vasculitis, SLE
Eyes	• Corneal arcus & xanthelasma	→ Hypercholesterolaemia

Examine upper or lower limbs as guided by history – may do both if history suggests a systemic problem

CORE EXAMINATION: UPPER LIMB

Component/action	Examine for	DD/potential findings/extra information
Inspection Expose SU, arms from shoulders • Colour • Size/symmetry • Venous pattern/appearance	• Pallor • Dusky • Unilateral swelling • Prominent veins • Skin lesion	→ Arterial occlusion → DVT → DVT, lymphoedema, cellulitis, malignancy → DVT → [see Appendix: Skin lesions]
Palpation • Temperature: use back of hands to assess temperature, feel full length of limb, compare side to side and distal to proximal • CRT: raise limb above heart level, press on distal phalanx of digit for 5 sec and release – time how long it takes for colour to return (should be <2 sec)	• Cold • Hot • Returns >2 seconds	→ Arterial insufficiency → Infection/inflammation; consider MSK cause → Arterial insufficiency/occlusion; consider cardiac causes
Pulses Move proximal to distal, compare directly side to side for symmetry and volume; grade 0–4+ [see notes 5] • Brachial: medial to the bicep tendon • Radial: between the radius and the flexor tendon on the bottom of the wrist	• Absent • Thready • Bounding	→ Arterial occlusion → Arterial insufficiency → Infection/inflammation; consider cardiac cause

PERIPHERAL VASCULAR

CORE EXAMINATION: LOWER LIMB

Component/action	Examine for	DD/potential findings/extra information
Inspection	• Colour • Size/symmetry • Superficial veins • Skin lesions	→ [see notes 1] → [see Appendix: Skin lesions]
Palpation • Temperature: use back of hands to assess temperature, feel full length of limb, compare side to side and distal to proximal • CRT: raise limb above heart level, press on distal phalanx of digit for 5 sec and release – time how long it takes for colour to return (should be <2 sec) • Palpate calves: palpate for oedema, with legs dependent, press for 5 sec over bony areas of shin, medial malleolus and dorsum of foot; grade 1–4 [see notes 4]	• Cold • Hot • Returns >2 seconds • Tenderness • Pitting	→ Arterial insufficiency/occlusion → Infection/inflammation; consider MSK cause → Arterial insufficiency/occlusion; consider cardiac causes → DVT (also MSK causes) → [see notes 3]
Pulses Move proximal to distal, compare directly side to side for symmetry and volume; grade 0–4+ [see notes 5] • Femoral: halfway between ASIS & pubic symphysis, below inguinal ligament • Popliteal: flex knee to 30°, ensure SU relaxed, grasp knee with both hands, thumbs in front, feel with fingers in popliteal fossa; often hard to feel; presence of more distal pulses reassures • Posterior tibial: behind medial malleolus • Dorsalis pedis: on dorsum of foot lateral to the extensor hallucis longus tendon	• Absent • Thready • Bounding	→ Arterial occlusion → Arterial insufficiency → Infection/inflammation; consider cardiac cause

ADDITIONAL EXAMINATION

Choose tests according to priority from a range of options (below) based on clinical reasoning – not necessary to do all

Cues from history / DDs / core examination	Component / action	Examine for	DD / potential findings / extra information
Infection or malignancy DD	**Axillary or inguinal lymph node examination [see Appendix: Lymph nodes for location]**	Lymphadenopathy [see Appendix: Lymph nodes] →	[see Appendix: Lymph nodes]
Onset of hypertension before 30 years of age Refractory hypertension	Auscultate renal arteries: superior and lateral to umbilicus bilaterally	• Bruits	→ Renal artery stenosis [see notes 2]
Decreased urination, peripheral oedema, SOB, nausea, weakness	Auscultate renal arteries: superior and lateral to umbilicus bilaterally	• Bruits	→ Acute renal failure secondary to renal artery stenosis [see notes 2]
Risk factors for vascular disease: smoking history, hypertension, hyperlipidaemia, diabetes mellitus, family history, PMH vascular events	Auscultate carotid arteries [see Cardiac], abdominal aorta (⅔ below xiphoid process above umbilicus), renal arteries (see above), femoral arteries (over femoral pulse); examine abdominal aorta (see below)	• Bruits	→ [see notes 2]
Symptoms of ischaemia: coldness in legs or feet, slow-healing wounds, colour changes in limbs, intermittent claudication	Auscultate abdominal aorta, renal, femoral arteries (see above)	• Bruits	→ [see notes 2]
Early signs of AAA: pulsating feeling in the abdomen, persistent back pain, pain in the abdomen, chest, lower back, or groin area OR Risk factors for AAA: older age, male sex, smoking, hypertension, coronary artery disease, first-degree relative with an AAA	Auscultate and examine AA Palpate deeply with two hands above umbilicus to identify pulsation of aorta; estimate width of aorta (should be <3 cm)	• Enlargement of AA • Bruits	→ May indicate an AAA or atherosclerosis, signalling a risk of aortic rupture or dissection → [see notes 2]

PERIPHERAL VASCULAR

CONCLUSION

Component / action	Examine for	DD / potential findings / extra information
Conclusion • Wash / gel hands • Thank SU, allow them to re-dress, check they are OK • Review observations (HR, BP, RR, SpO$_2$, temperature) • Decide on next steps with the SU or discuss & follow up once reviewed findings		Return to the aim of the examination – to localise the problem by: • Organising & correlating the history & test findings using clinical reasoning • Gathering sufficient information to allow more confident / directed action • Making a final list of DDs / concerns, in order of priority **Action** • Put together a reasoned / safe plan to cover all potential problems identified This could include: 1. Request further tests: e.g. Doppler if pulses not palpable, ankle / brachial pressure index to detect PAD vs. VI, USS / CT for sites of venous incompetence, narrowed or blocked arteries; measure calves if DVT is suspected, Wells score, D-dimer 2. Give advice / take appropriate action within scope 3. Make a referral / consult with MDT 4. Use safeguarding / gain a second opinion where uncertainty 5. Arrange a follow-up

1. Differences between venous and arterial insufficiency in lower limbs

		Venous insufficiency	Arterial insufficiency
History		• Varicose veins • DVTs	• Intermittent claudication • Rest pain
Inspection	Colour	• Brown discoloration (haemosiderosis)	• Pallor (ischaemia) • Mottling (acute ischaemia) • Redness with dependency (chronic ischaemia) • Black (tissue necrosis / gangrene)
	Oedema	• Often present	• Not normally present
	Skin changes	• Venous eczema • Atrophie blanche (white scar-like areas) • Inverted champagne bottle appearance to lower leg of lipodermatosclerosis	• Pale skin • Hairless • Onychogryphosis (thickened nails) • Fungal infections (skin / nails)
	Superficial veins	• Varicose veins in posterior lower leg (short saphenous) or medial leg and thigh (long saphenous) • Tenderness or warmth indicates superficial phlebitis	• Guttering of superficial veins (chronic arterial disease)
	Ulcers	• Gaiter area • Shallow edges • Exudate ++ • Mildly painful unless excessive oedema or infection	• On feet / toes / lateral malleolus • Punched-out appearance • Little exudate • Painful
Palpation	Temperature	• Warm	• Cold
	Capillary refill time	• <2 sec	• Increased in ischaemia • Reduced in dependent blood pooling
	Pulses	• Present	• Diminished or absent pulses

NOTES

2. Bruits

A bruit is an abnormal, audible vascular sound associated with turbulent blood flow through an artery, typically caused by partial obstruction, stenosis, or abnormal vessel structure. It is often heard during auscultation with a stethoscope and is most commonly associated with conditions like atherosclerosis or aneurysms.

Bruit	Significance
Carotid bruit [see Cardiac]	Indicates carotid artery stenosis, increasing the risk of stroke or TIA due to reduced blood flow to the brain
Renal artery bruit	Suggests renal artery stenosis, leading to hypertension and potential kidney dysfunction from reduced kidney blood flow
Abdominal aortic bruit	May indicate an AAA or atherosclerosis, signalling a risk of aortic rupture or dissection
Femoral bruit	Suggests PAD or femoral artery stenosis, leading to reduced blood flow to the legs, causing claudication (pain with walking)

3. DD Ankle swelling

Systems implicated: cardiovascular, respiratory, gastrointestinal, renal, endocrine, vascular

- Pitting oedema
  - Raised venous pressure
    - chronic venous insufficiency
    - right heart failure
    - volume overload (e.g. renal failure)
    - immobility
    - constrictive pericarditis
    - obesity (with associated Na^+/H_2O retention)
    - pregnancy
  - Reduced oncotic pressure (hypoalbuminaemia)
    - nephrotic syndrome
    - cirrhosis/liver failure
    - protein-losing enteropathy (e.g. IBD)
    - exfoliative dermatitis
  - Drug-related
    - calcium channel blockers
    - long-term corticosteroids
    - NSAIDs
- Non-pitting oedema
  - Lymphoedema
    - primary (e.g. Milroy's disease)
    - malignancy
    - filariasis
    - radiotherapy
    - lymph node clearance
  - Hypothyroidism
  - Pre-tibial myxoedema (Graves' disease)
- Unilateral/localised swelling
  - Acute DVT
  - Post-thrombotic syndrome
  - Associated with cellulitis

4. Grading oedema

0 – No oedema
1–2 mm depression, barely detectable: immediate rebound
2–4 mm deep pit: a few seconds to rebound
3–6 mm deep pit: 10–12 sec to rebound
4–8 mm deep pit: 20 sec to rebound

5. Grading pulses

Remember that some pulses are expected to be stronger or weaker than others, e.g. a femoral pulse may feel strong and a dorsalis pedis may feel weak, but this is expected therefore 2+.

4+   Bounding
3+   Increased
2+   Brisk, expected
1+   Diminished, weaker than expected
0   Absent, unable to palpate

NOTES

RESPIRATORY

WHY THIS SYSTEM?

Clues/correlations with history	Respiratory DDs
• SOB	Acute illness, e.g. URTI, pneumonia, PE Chronic lung disease, e.g. asthma, COPD, pulmonary fibrosis, bronchitis, cystic fibrosis Lung malignancy Consider cardiac cause
• Rib cage pain or discomfort when breathing/difficulty taking deep breaths	Acute trauma, rib #, pneumothorax, haemothorax, pneumonia, pleural effusion, pleurisy, PE Consider cardiac cause
• Productive cough or nasal mucus	Acute illness, e.g. URTI, pneumonia Exacerbation/flare of chronic illness, e.g. cystic fibrosis, COPD or smoking-related Consider ENT cause
• Unproductive/dry cough	Post-viral cough, URTI, asthma, allergenic sensitivity Consider ENT or GI cause
• Cough for more than 4 weeks ± haemoptysis	Covid, bronchitis, asthma, smoking-related, chronic infection, e.g. TB, lung cancer (rare) Consider GI or ENT cause
• Haemoptysis	Lung cancer, TB, pneumonia, chronic infection, chronic respiratory condition, PE Consider ENT cause
• Wheeze	Asthma, allergenic sensitivity, undiagnosed chronic lung disease, tumour
• Fatigue accompanying SOB	Anaemia, chronic lung disease, malignancy
• Reduced exercise tolerance: progressive/prolonged	Chronic respiratory disease
• Episodic, anxiety-induced SOB	Hyperventilation, asthma, anxiety
• History of injury involving thorax impact/potential thorax trauma	Rib #, pneumothorax, haemothorax
• History of long-haul travel/reduced mobility accompanying new onset SOB or calf swelling/pain	DVT – PE
• History inc. RoS that does **not** account for rapid onset SOB	PE
• Smoking history	Risk factor for interstitial lung disease & COPD
• Allergenic history with intermittent SOB/wheeze (potential correlation with animal/bird contact, pollutants or mould)	Asthma, allergenic sensitivity, lung hypersensitivity

! BEFORE starting the examination !

SU perspective: proactively explore any potential concerns beforehand

- Distress of being short of breath: start with an optimal, sustainable position to relieve effort during examination – forward sitting with legs on the floor & arms supported may be preferred over lying back on a bed
- Anxiety & difficulty of breathing:
  - Suggest to SU "*Can you slow down your breathing by blowing out gently & slowly through your mouth rather than trying to take deep breaths*" or alternatively "*Can you sigh out*"
  - Encourage diaphragmatic breathing (tummy breathing) – "*Put one hand on your tummy & feel it rise and fall*"
  - Encourage relaxation / distraction – "*Can you relax / drop your shoulders*" , "*Can you sigh out*" , "*Can you bring to mind a situation when you feel relaxed, such as being on holiday, or with your family perhaps*"
- Symptomatic relief prior to examination: oxygen, pain relief
- Concern for vulnerable exposure: explain the extent of exposure required, reassure about maintaining dignity, offer a chaperone
- Fear of worst case, e.g. lung cancer – acknowledge and reassure around the need for assessment to make an informed shared decision
- Minimise position changes if older adult / fatigue / SOB

RESPIRATORY

GENERAL INSPECTION

Component / action	Examine for	DD / potential findings / extra information
Introduction • Wash / gel hands • Introduce yourself, confirm SU, explain examination • Gain informed consent, explain ability to withdraw, stop the examination, decline specific tests or ask questions • Expose SU: top off, sitting in chair / on side of bed; use draping to expose only as required for each examination step		Consider a chaperone or ask "*Would you like to be supported by someone – is there someone in the waiting room?*" → Bra can be kept on as preferred in ♀
General appearance	• Unwell / distressed • Dyspnoea • Pain / discomfort breathing • Accessory muscle use • Pursed-lip breathing • Poor nutritional status / cachexia • Oxygen, drips, catheters, drains, medications	→ Consider position / comfort / medication to enable examination → Acute or chronic respiratory condition; consider cardiac cause → Acute trauma, rib #, pneumothorax, haemothorax, pneumonia, underlying inflammation, e.g. pleurisy, pleural effusion [see notes 1], PE → ↑ WOB, respiratory fatigue → Lower airway obstruction (usually COPD) → Wasting due to long-term ↑ respiratory effort, COPD, malignancy → e.g. inhalers, nebulisers
Respiration rate Count over 1 min whilst pretending to take pulse (below) Note rhythm, depth, and effort	• Tachypnoea – above 20 • Bradypnoea – below 12 + decreased GCS • Shallow / apical, erratic, effortful	→ Increased respiratory effort 2° to acute or chronic cause → Immediate medical attention required → ↑ WOB, respiratory fatigue, pain
Pulse rate: palpate radial pulse (time over 1 min) • Briefly assess volume	• Tachycardia • Bounding • Thready	→ Acute or chronic illness / distress / SOB, β_2-agonist Rx (e.g. salbutamol) → Hypercapnia, early sepsis [see **Cardiac**] → Severe respiratory compromise, late sepsis [see **Cardiac**]
Hands Inspect & feel for temperature Assess for flapping tremor: SU extends arms in front with wrists extended	• Peripheral cyanosis ± central cyanosis • Cold • Tar staining • Dilated veins • Fine physiological tremor • Irregular, jerky downward movement of the hands (asterixis)	→ Chronic respiratory disease, Raynaud's; consider PVS / cardiac cause – PVD / CCF → Pure peripheral cyanosis → Smoking → Hypercapnia → β_2-agonist Rx (e.g. salbutamol) → Respiratory failure (CO_2 retention); consider hepatic / renal failure

Nails	• Finger clubbing (look closely)	→ Chronic lung disease – interstitial/suppurative, malignancy [see notes 2 & 3]
	• Beau's lines	→ Prolonged or chronic illness
	• Koilonychia	→ Iron-deficiency anaemia
Face	• Cushingoid (moon face, plethora, acne, hirsute)	→ Long-term steroid Rx, e.g. for asthma, COPD, pulmonary fibrosis, CFA [see GI – Cushing's syndrome]
Eyes (gently pull down lower eyelid)	• Conjunctival pallor	→ Anaemia (cause of SOB)
Mouth (use a pen torch)	• Central cyanosis (blue lips & tongue)	→ Hypoxic lung disease; consider cardiac cause
	• Candida	→ Steroid inhalers, immunocompromised

Neck
• Inspect trachea position: ask SU to take a deep breath in
• Palpate – always warn SU beforehand: "*I'm going to feel for your windpipe*"
  ○ Place middle finger in suprasternal notch
  ○ Place second & ring fingers either side of the trachea
  ○ Note tracheal position
  ○ Ask SU to take a deep breath in, feeling for 'tug'
	• Scars, mass/lump
	
	• Tracheal deviation
	
	• Tug on inspiration
		→ Compression of upper airway, e.g. mass/malignancy/previous surgery scarring; consider thyroid examination [see Appendix: General lumps]
		→ Deviates towards collapse or away from tension, e.g. pneumothorax, pleural effusion
		→ ↑WOB, laryngomalacia (infants), hyperinflation (COPD)

RESPIRATORY

CORE EXAMINATION: THE THORAX

Component / action	Examine for	DD / potential findings / extra information
Complete steps below (as far as possible) for: • Posterior: SU sitting in chair / on side of bed, arms crossed in front / to opposite shoulders if SU able • Anterior: reposition SU supported in chair / in bed supine at 45°		→ Begin here to access greater surface area / findings → Ensure comfort & increased support where possible; consider SU may want to sit up / lean forward for position of ease
Inspection • Briefly expose & observe entire thorax noting shape from front / side / behind • Using draping, inspect skin, muscle bulk & ribs in more detail	• Increased A–P diameter • Deformity of chest / spine • Intercostal indrawing (Hoover's sign) • Bony deformities, bruises • Masses • Scars, sinus tracts • Gynaecomastia / interscapular fat pad (buffalo hump)	→ Hyperinflation (COPD) → Pectus excavatum, pectus carinatum (asthma), scoliosis → ↑WOB, respiratory fatigue (common in unwell infants), hyperinflation in chronic respiratory disease, e.g. COPD → Acute trauma, rib #, potential pneumothorax → Malignancy → Thoracotomy (lobectomy / pneumonectomy), old chest drain sites → Long-term steroid Rx, e.g. in asthma, COPD, pulmonary fibrosis, CFA [see GI – Cushing's syndrome]

Palpation
• Assess symmetry of expansion
  ○ Place both hands at level of 10th rib, thumbs touching, fingers resting upwards
  ○ Ask SU "*Take a deep breath*"
  ○ Observe your thumb movements for symmetry
 	
• Intercostal spaces & ribs for areas of tenderness or evidence of bony injury
 	
• Tactile fremitus
  ○ Ask SU "*Say 'blue balloons' each time I put my hands on your chest*"
  ○ Use ball / ulnar surface of hands to feel vibrations throughout lung zones [see notes 4 & 5]
	• Asymmetrical expansion
	
	• Pain / tenderness
	
	• Increased fremitus
	• Reduced fremitus
	
	• Normal or reduced fremitus
		→ Collapse, e.g. pneumothorax, atelectasis
		→ Lobectomy / pneumonectomy 2° to Ca, bronchiectasis, trauma, TB
		→ Consolidation, e.g. pneumonia
		▶ Pleural effusion
		NB. Large degree of asymmetry may be obvious on inspection
		→ Acute trauma, rib #, muscle strain, underlying inflammation, e.g. pleurisy
		
		→ Consolidation, mass, inflammatory exudate, pus
		→ Hyperinflation (COPD), pleural effusion, pneumothorax, obstructive atelectasis / collapse
		→ Compressive collapse

Percussion • Start in supraspinous / supraclavicular fossae & work down chest • Compare side to side throughout lung zones [see notes 6 for points of percussion] • Map out any abnormalities in percussion note	• Hyperresonance • Dull • Dull at bases • Stony dull	→ Hyperinflation (COPD), pneumothorax → Consolidation, collapse → Pulmonary oedema (HF) → Pleural effusion

Auscultation

Place stethoscope directly on skin; if clothing in place, lift clothing to place stethoscope

- Instruct SU to breathe normally through mouth → Specifying mouth avoids noisy nasal breathing
- Start in supraspinous/supraclavicular fossae & work down chest
- Compare side to side throughout lung zones [**see notes 7** for points of auscultation]
- Map out any abnormalities, listening for breath sound presence, character & added noises [**see notes 8**]

- Breath sounds (normal = vesicular)
- Bronchial (excl. over trachea/major bronchi) → Consolidation

Added sounds:
- Wheeze → Narrowing/obstruction of airways, asthma, COPD, tumour
- Crepitations/crackles
  - Coarse → Fluid in air spaces: secretions, pus, oedema → Pneumonia, suppurative lung disease, e.g. bronchiectasis, cystic fibrosis
  - Fine → Pulmonary oedema (at bases), COPD, interstitial lung disease, e.g. pulmonary fibrosis

- If crepitations heard, ask SU to cough & listen again
  - Clears with cough → Normal secretions or URTI
  - Pleural rub → Pleural inflammation, e.g. pleurisy, PE

ADDITIONAL EXAMINATION

Choose tests according to priority from a range of options (below) based on clinical reasoning – not necessary to do all

Cues from history/DDs/core examination	Component/action	Examine for	DD/potential findings/extra information
Infection or malignancy DD	Head and neck and axillary lymph node examination [**see Appendix: Lymph nodes for location**]	Lymphadenopathy [**see Appendix: Lymph nodes**] →	[**see Appendix: Lymph nodes**]
PE DD	**JVP** • SU at 45°, head turned slightly to their left • Use tangential lighting to highlight contours and subtle pulsations • Don't turn head too far – you want neck muscles to relax • Look for double pulsation on left side of neck • Estimate height above sternal angle in cm • Normally <3–4 cm, if raised can measure [**see Cardiac notes 1**]	• Prominent IJV extending higher by 3–4 cm above the sternal angle • Kussmaul's sign (rises with inspiration) →	PE, SVC obstruction; consider cardiac causes [**see Cardiac**]

RESPIRATORY

RESPIRATORY

CONCLUSION

Component / action	Examine for	DD / potential findings / extra information
Conclusion • Wash / gel hands • Thank SU, allow them to re-dress, check they are OK • Review observations (HR, BP, RR, SpO$_2$, temperature) • See sputum pot if appropriate • Decide on next steps with the SU or discuss & follow up once findings reviewed		Return to the aim of the examination – to localise the problem by: • Organising & correlating the history & test findings using clinical reasoning [**see notes 9**] • Gathering sufficient information to allow more confident / directed action • Making a final list of DDs / concerns, in order of priority Action • Put together a reasoned / safe plan to cover all potential problems identified This could include: 1. Request further tests – sputum sample, peak flow, PFR, ABG, CXR 2. Give advice / take appropriate action within scope 3. Make a referral / consult with MDT 4. Use safeguarding / gain a second opinion where any uncertainty 5. Arrange a follow-up

1. DD Pleural effusion
- Exudative: due to inflammation/increased capillary permeability (high protein content >30g/L)
  - Infection
    - Pneumonia
    - TB
  - Infarction (pulmonary)
    - PE*
  - Inflammation
    - RA
    - SLE
    - Pancreatitis
  - Malignancy
    - Bronchogenic
    - Mesothelioma
    - Breast
- Transudative: due to increased hydrostatic pressure/low plasma oncotic pressure (low protein content <30g/L)
  - HF, LVF
  - Volume overload
  - PE*
  - Liver cirrhosis
  - Nephrotic syndrome
  - Hypoalbuminaemia
  - Pericarditis
  - Meigs' syndrome (triad: benign ovarian tumour, ascites, pleural effusion)

*NB. PE can cause either

2. DD Interstitial lung disease (pulmonary fibrosis)
1. Idiopathic
   - Idiopathic pulmonary fibrosis/cryptogenic fibrosing alveolitis (different names for same condition)
2. Due to inhaled antigen (i.e. EAA)
   - Bird fancier's lung
   - Farmer's lung
3. Due to inhaled irritant
   - Asbestosis
   - Silicosis
   - Coal worker's pneumoconiosis
4. Associated with systemic disease
   - SLE
   - RA
   - Sarcoid
   - Systemic sclerosis
5. Iatrogenic
   - Methotrexate
   - Amiodarone
   - Radiotherapy

3. Features of finger clubbing
- Increased fluctuance of nailbed
- Loss of nailbed angle
- Increased longitudinal curvature of nail
- Drumsticking

DD Finger clubbing
- Respiratory disease
  - Interstitial lung disease
  - Pulmonary fibrosis
  - Pneumonitis inc. hypersensitivity
  - Sarcoidosis
  - Bronchiolitis
  - Alveolitis
  - Vasculitis
  - Suppurative lung disease
    - Bronchiectasis (pus in the tubes)
    - Abscess (pus in a collection)
    - Empyema (pus outside the lung)
    - Cystic fibrosis (pus everywhere)
  - Malignancy
    - Bronchogenic carcinoma
    - Mesothelioma
- Other causes [see also Cardiac and GI]
  - Thyroid acropachy (Graves' disease)
  - Familial

NOTES

4. Lung anatomy & landmarks: anterior (A); posterior (B); lateral (C)

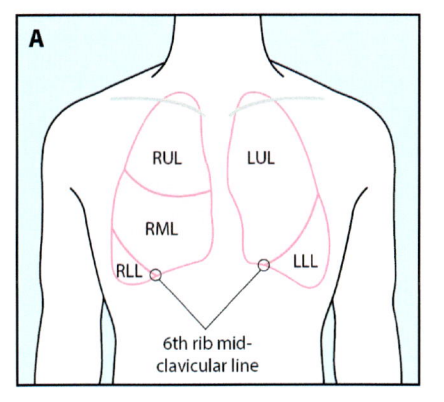
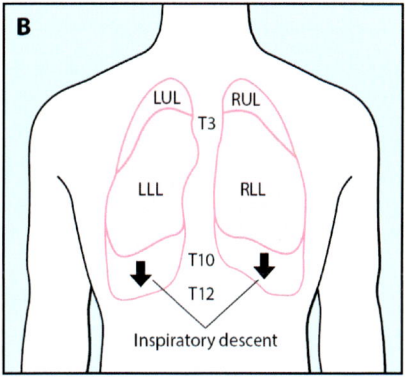
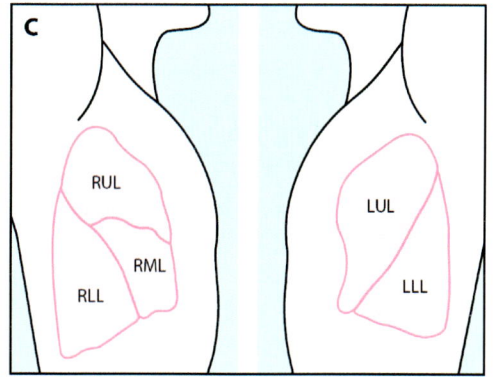

5. Tactile fremitus hand placement

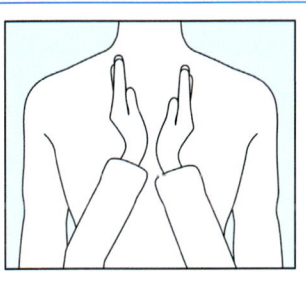
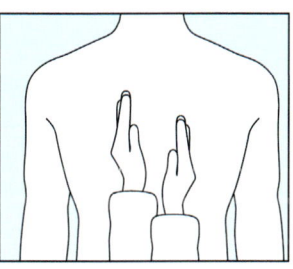
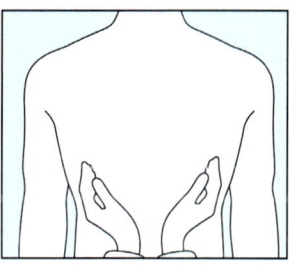

6. Percussion and auscultation points

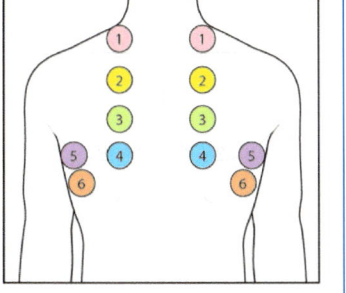
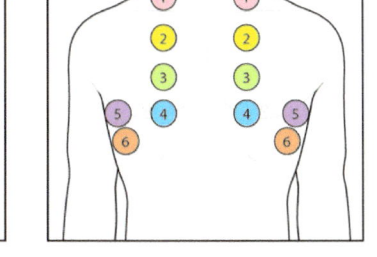

NOTES

7. Breath / added sounds – characteristics & features

Breath / added sound	Description	Location normally heard	Length / features
Bronchial breathing	• Loud & blowing	• Over trachea / major bronchi (manubrium) • If in the peripheries = abnormal / areas of consolidation	• Expiration > inspiration • Audible gap between inspiration & expiration
Vesicular breathing	• Soft, low pitch	• Over most of both lungs	• Inspiration > expiration • No pause between inspiration & expiration
Coarse crackles	• Loud, lower-pitched, longer-duration 'bubbling' or 'gurgling' sound	• Varies	• Early to mid-inspiration • May occur on expiration too
Fine crackles	• Soft, high-pitched, brief 'popping' or 'rubbing hair between fingers' sound	• Varies	• Mid to late inspiration
Wheeze	• High-pitched, musical, continuous sound (like a whistle)	• Varies	• Most often heard on expiration, but can be inspiratory if severe
Pleural rub	• Harsh, dry, grating or creaking / squeaking	• Usually confined to specific area of chest wall	• Inspiration & expiration
Stridor	• Loud, high-pitched, 'shrill' • Indicates significant airway narrowing & medical emergency	• Heard without stethoscope • Loudest over neck	• Inspiration / expiration or both

8. Correlation of findings table

	Normal lung	Consolidation/mass e.g. pneumonia/malignancy	Collapse* e.g. obstructive atelectasis (bronchus blocked)	Pleural effusion**	Pneumothorax	Hyperinflation e.g. COPD
Mediastinal shift	Nil	Nil	Towards	Away if large	Away if tension	Nil
Tactile fremitus	Normal	↑	↓ or absent. NB. If bronchus is open, some vibrations may still transmit, e.g. with compressive collapse	↓ or absent	↓ or absent	↓
Percussion note	Resonant	Dull	Dull	Stony dull	(Hyper)resonant	Hyperresonant
Auscultation breath sounds	Vesicular Bronchial over trachea/major bronchi	Bronchial or ↓	↓ or absent	↓ or absent	↓ or absent	↓

*Lobectomy/pneumonectomy
- Examination findings identical to collapse
- Given away by thoracotomy scar on chest, but some examiners will hide this to test you
- Indications: bronchogenic Ca (25% of non-SCLC is resectable), bronchiectasis, trauma, TB

**Raised hemidiaphragm
- Examination findings identical to effusion
- CXR to differentiate
- Due to phrenic nerve palsy
- Caused by thoracic surgery/trauma/malignancy

NOTES

APPENDICES

LYMPH NODES

Systematic palpation of the lymph nodes helps identify any enlarged or abnormal lymph nodes, which can be a sign of infection, inflammation, or malignancy. Assess an enlarged lymph node as you would any other lump [see **Appendix: General lumps**].

Component / action	Examine for	DD / potential findings / extra information
Use draping to expose only as required for each examination step Position SU as appropriate to facilitate relaxation of musculature **Inspection** Inspect relevant lymph node areas [**see notes 1**]	• Swelling • Erythema • Asymmetry	→ Lymphadenopathy – reactive or infectious, malignancy → Inflammation or infection, e.g. lymphadenitis → Localised infection or inflammation, malignancy, unilateral reactive node, e.g. insect bite
Palpation • Use a systematic approach [**see notes 4–6**] • Using finger pads of two or three fingers, move in circular motion with light touch, palpating the full chain in each location	• Size • Consistency • Tenderness • Heat • Immobility	→ [**see notes 2 & 3**]

1. Drainage of lymph nodes

System	Relevant node(s)	Key area drained
Cardiac	Axillary (indirect)	Chest wall, breast
ENT	Head & neck	Ear, nose, throat, sinuses, tonsils
Gastrointestinal	Inguinal, supraclavicular, head & neck	Anal canal, genitalia (inguinal); mouth, pharynx (head & neck); stomach, pancreas, colon (supraclavicular)
Musculoskeletal	Axillary, inguinal	Upper & lower limbs, joints, skin
Neurological	Head & neck	Scalp, meninges, cranial regions
Peripheral vascular	Axillary, inguinal	Upper & lower limb vasculature
Respiratory	Head & neck, axillary	Upper airway (head & neck); chest wall/lower airway (axillary)

NOTES

2. Typical characteristics of lymphadenopathy
- Healthy lymph nodes are not palpable or may feel small & firm
- Painful, soft, mobile, tender – reactive or infectious lymphadenitis
- Firm, rubbery, non-tender – mobile – lymphoma
- Hard, fixed, non-tender – metastatic carcinoma
- Matted nodes – tuberculosis or sarcoidosis

3. DD Lymphadenopathy
1. Localised
   - Acute local infection (e.g. tonsillitis)
   - Neoplastic
     - Local malignancy
     - Solitary distant metastasis
2. Generalised
   - Acute generalised infection
     - HIV seroconversion
   - Chronic infection
     - TB 'cold abscesses'
     - Syphilis
     - HIV
   - Neoplastic
     - Multiple distant metastases
     - Haematological
     - Lymphoma
     - CLL
   - Systemic disease
     - Sarcoidosis
     - RA

4. Head & neck
Position SU sitting. Lower neckline of garment. Relax sternomastoid muscles by asking SU to tip head forward for deep cervical nodes. Use a systematic approach, move proximal to distal, following drainage pattern (1–9 in diagram), bilaterally at the same time where possible.

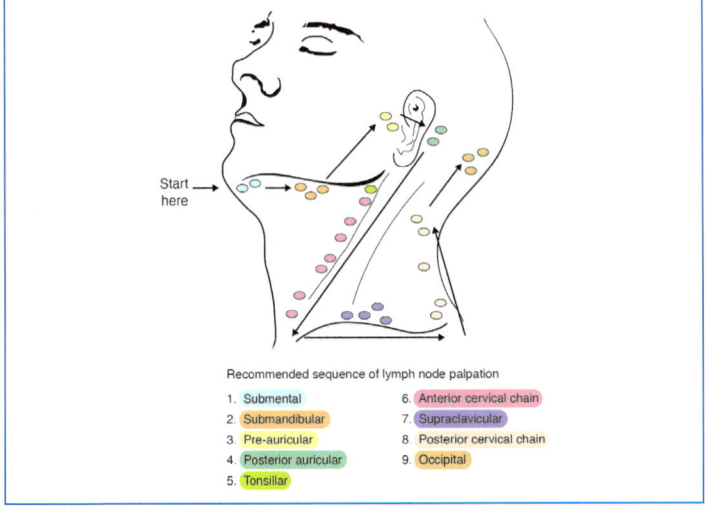

Recommended sequence of lymph node palpation

1. Submental
2. Submandibular
3. Pre-auricular
4. Posterior auricular
5. Tonsillar
6. Anterior cervical chain
7. Supraclavicular
8. Posterior cervical chain
9. Occipital

- Pre-auricular: drain eyelids and forehead
- Posterior auricular: drain scalp and ear
- Occipital: drain scalp
- Submental: drain lower lip, chin, tip of tongue
- Submandibular: drain cheeks, upper lip, tongue, gums
- Tonsillar: drain tonsils and pharynx
- Anterior cervical chain: drain superficial neck, pharynx, larynx, tonsils, thyroid
- Posterior cervical chain: drain posterior scalp and neck, skin of upper back, auricle
- Supraclavicular: drain thoracic cavity, abdomen (left side), arm and chest wall (right side)

5. Axillary

Position SU supine at 45°. SU places arm behind head to relax musculature. Drape to expose axilla, cover chest (e.g. gown removed from one arm at a time). Use a systematic approach, move proximal to distal following drainage pattern (1–5 in diagram).

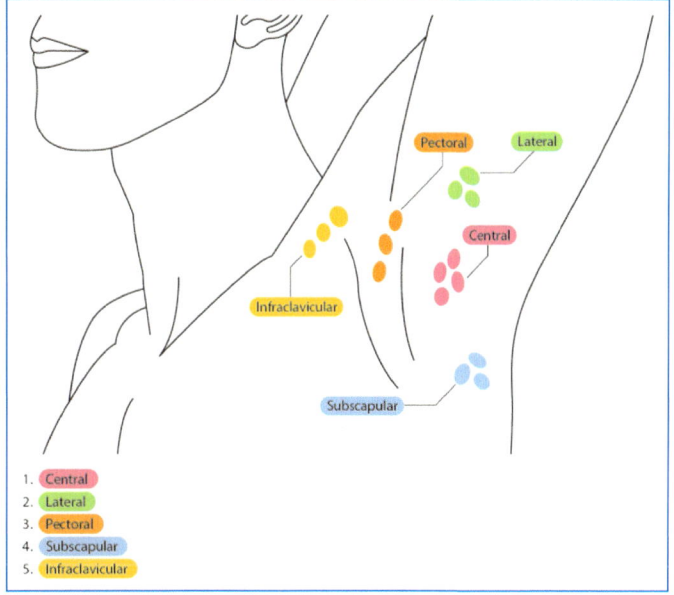

- Central: drain from pectoral, subscapular and lateral nodes
- Lateral: drain upper limb and lateral breast
- Pectoral: drain anterior thoracic wall and breast
- Subscapular: drain posterior thoracic wall and scapular region
- Infraclavicular: drain upper lateral arm and pectoral region

6. Inguinal

Position SU supine. Drape to expose inguinal areas and cover genitalia (e.g. gown between legs). Use a systematic approach, move proximal to distal (medial to lateral).

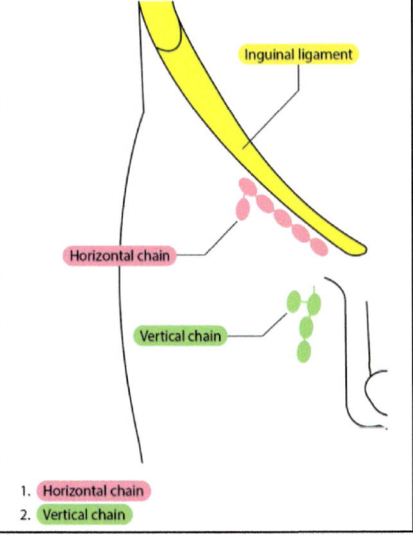

- **Horizontal chain (superficial):** drain lower abdomen, external genitalia, perineum, anal canal, and superficial buttocks
- **Vertical chain (lateral):** drain from superficial chain, thigh and leg (deep structures), glans penis, upper vagina, cervix, and perineum

GENERAL EXAMINATION OF A LUMP

This sequence can be used to assess any lump, swelling or protrusion. Tailored examination of lumps in specific areas is covered in the subsequent tables: thyroid/neck lump, breast lump, scrotal swelling. The examination should also include examination of regional lymph nodes [**see Appendix: Lymph nodes**].

! BEFORE starting the examination !

SU perspective: proactively explore any potential concerns beforehand
• Concern for vulnerable exposure depending on location of lump: explain the extent of exposure required, reassure about maintaining dignity, offer a chaperone • Anxiety that this may be a sign of malignancy: explain importance of moving through a series of checks together to help guide what to do next/who to refer to, to move forward with support • Any history of sexual abuse/trauma – trauma-informed approach – put the SU in control

GENERAL LUMP EXAMINATION

Component / action	Examine for	DD / potential findings / extra information
Use draping to expose only as required for each examination step **Inspection**: from front & side • Note relationship to surrounding anatomical structures **[see notes 1]** • Measure size in two dimensions, shape, colour, contour • Overlying skin	• Scars • Erythema • Pigmented • Punctum • Discharge	→ Previous surgery, e.g. thyroidectomy, lymph node biopsy / excision, radiotherapy-related scarring → Inflammation / infection → Melanoma **[see Appendix: Skin lesions]** → Typical of sebaceous cyst → Abscess
Palpation: "*Tell me if you feel any discomfort*"; compare with other side of body (if applicable) • Consistency • Mobility (moving lump in two planes, observing for skin wrinkling) • Ask SU to assume a position that contracts the underlying musculature – try to move lump; if suspicious of a ganglion, ask SU to move joint that involves that particular tendon & feel if lump moves too • Fluctuance (hold the lump on opposite sides, press downwards with one finger) • Temperature • Pulsatility • Tenderness • Borders • Reducibility • Compressibility	• Soft • Hard • Rubbery • Tethered • Fluid- / fat-filled • Increased warmth • Pulsations • Tender • Regular • Irregular • Ill-defined • Reducible – disappears when pressed & does not return spontaneously • Emptied by pressure but reappears spontaneously upon release	→ Cyst / lipoma → Suspicious for malignancy → Lymph node **[see Appendix: Lymph nodes]** → Suspicious for malignancy, ganglion cyst → Cyst, hydrocoele, lipoma → Inflammation / infection → Vascular origin, e.g. aneurysm → Inflammation / infection → Likely benign, e.g. lipoma / cyst → Suspicious for malignancy → Inflammation / suspicious for malignancy → **[see hernia examination below]** → Vascular, e.g. varicose vein
Palpation of regional lymph nodes **[see Appendix: Lymph nodes]**	• Lymphadenopathy	→ **[see Appendix: Lymph nodes]**
Auscultate	• Bruits • Bowel sounds	→ Goitre / aneurysm → See hernia examination below
Transilluminate with pen torch: apply light across the lump	• 'Glowing'	→ Fluid-filled, e.g. cyst, hydrocoele, or fat-filled, e.g. lipoma

THYROID / NECK LUMP EXAMINATION

Component / action	Examine for	DD / potential findings / extra information
General appearance	• Underweight, fidgety, tremulous, sweaty, flushed, restless • Overweight, warmly dressed, hair loss, dry skin, deep voice	→ Hyperthyroidism [see notes 2.8] → Hypothyroidism [see notes 2.4]
Hands & wrist Radial pulse rate, time over 1 min	• Acropachy (clubbing) • Palmar erythema • Fine tremor • Tachycardia • Bradycardia	→ Graves' disease [see notes 2.6] → Hyperthyroid → Hyperthyroid → Hyperthyroid → Hypothyroid
Face	• Flushed • Thin brittle eyebrows	→ Hyperthyroid → Hypothyroid
Eyes "*Follow my finger; tell me if you see double*" then slowly move a pen in an H-pattern in front of SU (approx. arm's length from face) Move finger upwards to see lid retract; quickly move finger downwards to look for delay in lids descending	• Exophthalmos • Ophthalmoplegia (esp. upward gaze) • Eyelid lag	→ Graves' disease [see notes 2.7] → Graves' disease → Hyperthyroid
Limbs • Reflexes [see **General neurology**] • Muscle power testing [see **General neurology**]	• Brisk • Slow • Proximal myopathy (shoulder ABduction, hip girdle strength)	→ Hyperthyroid → Hypothyroid → Hyperthyroid
Inspection of thyroid: from front & sides • Location • Ask SU to protrude tongue	• Midline, anterior / posterior triangle [see notes 2.2] • Upward movement of thyroid	→ Narrows DD [see notes 2.1] → Thyroglossal cyst

APPENDIX: GENERAL LUMPS

Palpation
- Ask the patient to relax their neck muscles
- Place your fingers just below the cricoid cartilage
- Use both hands to gently palpate the thyroid lobes & isthmus
- Ask the patient to swallow again while palpating – feel for upward movement
- Palpate the lymph nodes of the head & neck [see Appendix: Lymph nodes]

Auscultate
- For bruit (turbulent blood flow through the thyroid arteries) [see PVS notes]

• Diffuse enlargement (goitre) [see notes 2.3]	→	Graves' disease (hyperthyroidism), Hashimoto's thyroiditis (hypothyroidism)
• Asymmetry	→	Single nodule enlargement; thyroid adenoma (benign), thyroid carcinoma (esp. if hard, fixed, irregular, or rapidly growing)
• Thrill	→	Graves' disease
• Soft	→	Simple goitre
• Firm / rubbery	→	Hashimoto's thyroiditis
• Hard	→	Malignancy
• Widespread irregularity	→	Multinodular goitre [see notes 2.5]
• Immobility	→	Malignancy
• Asymmetrical elevation	→	Unilateral thyroid mass
• Lymphadenopathy	→	[see Appendix: Lymph nodes]
• Bruit	→	Graves' disease most commonly

134

BREAST LUMP EXAMINATION

Component / action	Examine for	DD / potential findings / extra information
• Expose SU to waist • Position SU sitting upright • Ask SU to identify location of lump & ask if painful		Consider a chaperone or ask *"Would you like to be supported by someone – is there someone in the waiting room?"*

Inspection
• Hands on thighs (pectoral muscles relaxed)
• Hands pressing into hips (pectoral muscles contracted) accentuates puckering; if mass moves suggests tethering
• Hands behind head leaning forward (accentuates asymmetry, skin dimpling, puckering)
	• Scars – breast & axilla
	• Asymmetry
	
	• Masses – obvious lump
	
	• Nipple abnormalities
	  ○ Inversion
	
	  ○ Discharge
	  ○ Scaly skin
	  ○ Erythema
	  ○ Puckering
	  ○ Peau d'orange (dimpling)
		→ Mastectomy, lumpectomy, biopsy
		→ Obvious differences – asymmetry in size may be normal; check with SU
		→ Malignant / benign [see notes 3.1]
		
		→ Malignancy, mastitis, breast abscess (can be normal; check with SU)
		→ Mastitis, malignancy
		→ Paget's disease of the nipple (intraductal carcinoma)
		→ Infection, mastitis, malignancy
		→ Malignancy
		→ Inflammatory breast cancer [see notes 3.3]

Palpation Position SU supine at 45° hand behind head on side being examined; start with unaffected side • Use pads of 3 middle fingers • View the breast as a clock face & examine each 'hour' from the outside towards the nipple • Palpate axillary tail • Palpate nipple, ask SU to express discharge if appropriate • Palpate lymph nodes of the axilla and the supraclavicular nodes [see Appendix: Lymph nodes]	• Breast mass • Milky discharge • Purulent discharge • Blood-stained discharge • Lymphadenopathy	→ Malignant / benign [see notes 3.1] → Prolactinoma (non-puerperal lactation) → Mastitis, breast abscess → Ductal carcinoma *in situ* → [see Appendix: Lymph nodes]

SCROTAL SWELLING EXAMINATION

Component / action	Examine for	DD / potential findings / extra information
• Expose SU: remove underwear • Position SU lying flat with one pillow • Ask SU to identify location of lump & ask if painful		Consider a chaperone or ask *"Would you like to be supported by someone – is there someone in the waiting room?"*
Inspection • Ask SU to move penis to allow inspection of scrotum & perineum	• Scars • Masses • Swelling • Erythema • Skin lesions	⟶ Previous surgery, e.g. vasectomy ⟶ Malignancy [**see notes 4.1 & 4.4**], perineal abscess ⟶ Hydrocoele ⟶ Cellulitis, fungal infection ⟶ e.g. warts (human papillomavirus) [**see Appendix: Skin lesions**]
Palpation • Testicles • Examine normal testicle first; palpate testis with both hands between thumb & index finger; assess if lump part of testicle or separate from it • Epididymis & spermatic cord • Palpate inguinal lymph nodes [**see Appendix: Lymph nodes**]	• Hard mass • 'Bag of worms' • Tenderness [**see notes 4.2**] • Cough impulse (see additional tests) • Unable to identify top of lump • Tenderness • Mass • Tenderness • Lymphadenopathy	⟶ Malignancy, epididymo-orchitis ⟶ Varicocoele [**see notes 4.3**] ⟶ Epididymo-orchitis ⟶ Inguinal hernia or varicocoele ⟶ Inguinal hernia [**see Examination of hernia**] ⟶ Epididymitis, e.g. chlamydia ⟶ Spermatocoele ⟶ Epididymitis, prostatitis ⟶ [**see Appendix: Lymph nodes**]
• Transillumination with pen torch: apply light source across the lump	• 'Glowing'	⟶ Hydrocoele

APPENDIX: GENERAL LUMPS

EXAMINATION OF HERNIA

Component/action	Examine for	DD/ potential findings/Extra information
Ask SU in which position the swelling is most obvious: sitting, standing, supine and then examine in this position • "Can you show me where you have you noticed the abnormality?" • "Is it painful?"		Consider a chaperone or ask "Would you like to be supported by someone – is there someone in the waiting room?"
Inspection (both sides if appropriate) • Measure size in two dimensions • Anatomical location	• Groin • Umbilicus • Midline abdomen • Lateral anterior abdomen	→ Inguinal/femoral hernia → Umbilical/paraumbilical hernia → Epigastric/incisional hernia → Spigelian hernia
• Overlying/surrounding skin	• Scars • Erythema	→ Incisional hernia → Strangulated hernia
• Cough impulse: ask SU to "Give me a loud cough"	• Expansile impulse seen over the swelling	→ Positive cough impulse – likely hernia → Negative cough impulse – incarcerated hernia [see notes 5.2], lymph node [see Appendix: Lymph nodes], cyst, lipoma [see Appendix: General lump examination]
Palpation • Location [see notes 5.4]	• Hernia above pubic tubercle • Hernia below pubic tubercle	→ Indirect/direct inguinal hernia → Femoral hernia
• Consistency • Temperature • Cough impulse: ask SU to "Give me a loud cough"	• Tense skin • Warm • Expansile impulse felt over the swelling	→ Incarcerated hernia → Incarcerated hernia → Positive cough impulse – likely hernia → Negative cough impulse – incarcerated hernia, lymph node, cyst, lipoma
• Reducibility: ask SU "Can you push the lump back inside?"	• Reducible • Irreducible	→ Hernia → Strangulated hernia
• Palpate scrotum in ♂	• Swelling extends into scrotum (cannot get 'above' scrotal swelling)	→ Indirect inguinal hernia
• Palpate inguinal and left supraclavicular lymph nodes [see Appendix: Lymph nodes]	• Lymphadenopathy	→ [see Appendix: Lymph nodes]
Auscultate hernia	• Bowel sounds	→ Herniated bowel or omentum

Examination of a lump may then be followed by further tests to assist in making a diagnosis. These might include imaging (usually ultrasound), biopsy for microbiology &/or histology, blood test for inflammatory or tumour markers.

1. General lumps notes
Lumps in relation to anatomical location

Anatomical location	Type of lump	Mobility	Relation to surrounding structures	Other features
Skin (epidermis / dermis)	Epidermoid (sebaceous) cyst	Fixed to skin, mobile over deeper tissue	Tethered to skin	Central punctum, dome-shaped, may rupture
	Dermatofibroma	Firm, fixed to skin	Skin puckers on compression (dimple sign)	Often pigmented or pink
Subcutaneous tissue	Lipoma	Freely mobile in all directions	Not attached to skin or deep structures	Soft, lobulated, non-tender
Joint capsule / tendon sheath	Ganglion cyst	Fixed to deep structures, not to skin	Arises near joints / tendons	Cystic, transilluminates, non-tender
Peripheral nerve	Neuroma / schwannoma	Mobile side-to-side, not along nerve path	Along course of nerve	Tinel's sign may be positive
Blood vessel	Aneurysm / vascular lump	Pulsatile, may expand with Valsalva	In continuity with artery or vein	Bruit on auscultation
Bone / periosteum	Osteochondroma	Immobile	Fixed to bone, often protrudes from surface	Hard, usually painless
	Bone tumour / sarcoma	Immobile	Deep, fixed to bone, may distort overlying tissues	Hard, may be malignant
Fascia / muscle	Desmoid tumour	May be fixed to underlying fascia	Deep-seated, infiltrative	Rare, locally aggressive
Lymphatic tissue (nodes)	Reactive lymph node	Soft, mobile	Not tethered to surrounding structures	Tender, often recent infection
	Malignant lymph node	Firm / hard, may be fixed	May invade adjacent tissues	Non-tender, persistent

NOTES

APPENDIX: GENERAL LUMPS NOTES

Common benign lumps

	Lipoma	Sebaceous cyst	Ganglion
Description	Benign fatty tumour	Epidermal proliferation within dermis	Degenerative cyst from synovum of joint/tendon
Common sites	Anywhere fat can expand (*not scalp or palms*)	Anywhere on body (most common on trunk, neck, face & scalp)	Dorsum of hand/wrist Dorsal foot
Depth	Subcutaneous	Intradermal	Subcutaneous
Other features	Smooth Imprecise margins Fluctuant	Central punctum	Moves with tendon May transilluminate
Complications	Symptoms 2° to pressure effects Malignant change (*very rare*)	Infection common	Rare
Management	Conservative Excision for cosmetic reasons or local pressure effects	Incision & drainage if infected Occasionally antibiotics needed Non-infected cysts can be 'shelled out' under local anaesthesia	Conservative (50% disappear) Aspiration Excision

NOTES

Red flag signs for a lump

Red flag	Why it's concerning
Hard, fixed (non-mobile) lump	Suggests possible malignancy (cancer invading tissues)
Rapid growth	Fast-growing masses are more suspicious of aggressive tumours
Size >2 cm (especially if growing)	Larger lumps have a higher risk of being malignant
Irregular or poorly-defined borders	Benign lumps are usually smooth; irregular borders suggest invasion
Persistent pain (especially deep, aching)	Can indicate nerve invasion or aggressive behaviour
Systemic symptoms (e.g. unexplained weight loss, fever, night sweats)	'B symptoms' – often associated with lymphoma or systemic malignancy
Skin changes over a lump (ulceration, dimpling, colour change)	Skin involvement suggests possible malignancy or severe infection
History of cancer	Any new lump in someone with prior cancer is concerning for metastasis
Non-resolving over 4–6 weeks	Benign/reactive lumps usually shrink; persistent lumps need investigation

2. Thyroid notes
2.1. DD Neck lump
- Midline
  - Goitre
  - Thyroglossal cyst
- Anterior triangle
  - Branchial cyst – under the top of SCM
  - Carotid body tumour
  - Lymph node [see lymph nodes]
- Posterior triangle
  - Cystic hygroma (above clavicle)
  - Lymph node
- Anywhere
  - Sebaceous cyst
  - Lipoma

2.2. The anterior and posterior triangles of the neck

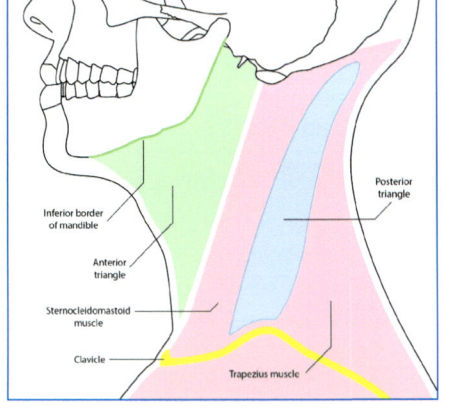

NOTES

2.3. DD Goitre
- Multinodular goitre
- Graves' disease
- Solitary nodule (adenoma/carcinoma)
- Hashimoto's thyroiditis
- Subacute thyroiditis

2.4. DD Hypothyroidism
- Autoimmune
  - Primary atrophic thyroiditis (no goitre)
  - Hashimoto's initially
- Acquired
  - Iodine deficiency (no. 1 cause worldwide)
  - Subacute thyroiditis
  - Iatrogenic
    - Surgery
    - Radioiodine
    - Carbimazole
    - Lithium
    - Amiodarone
- Secondary
  - Panhypopituitarism (very rare)

2.5. Multinodular goitre (MNG)
- Most common large goitre
- Rarely can be smooth rather than multinodular to feel
- SU usually euthyroid = non-toxic MNG
- Hyperthyroid = toxic MNG
- Indications for surgery in non-toxic MNG
  - Cosmetic reasons
  - Local compression effect

2.6. Graves' disease
- Classic features
  - Goitre
  - Thyrotoxicosis
  - Eye disease (50%)
    - Exophthalmos*
    - Ophthalmoplegia*
  - Pretibial myxoedema*
  - Thyroid acropachy*
    - *unique to Graves'*
- Factors differentiating from toxic MNG
  - Smooth goitre (MNG rarely smooth)
  - Graves'-unique features as above
  - TSH-receptor antibodies
- Indications for surgery
  - Cosmetic reasons
  - Local compression effect
  - Failed medical Rx
  - Intolerant of medication

2.7. A note on thyroid eye signs
- Any cause of hyperthyroidism
  - Lid retraction
  - Lid lag
- Specific to Graves' disease
  - Exophthalmos
  - Ophthalmoplegia

2.8. DD Hyperthyroidism
- Graves' disease
- Toxic MNG } 90%
- Toxic nodule (usually adenoma)
- Thyroiditis in the initial phase
  - Hashimoto's
  - Post-partum
  - Subacute
- Secondary (*rare*)
  - TSHoma
  - Hydatidiform mole
  - Choriocarcinoma

NOTES

3. Breast lump notes

3.1. DD Breast lump
- Malignant (invasive ductal carcinoma most common)
- Benign
  - Fibroadenoma
  - Breast cyst (may be painful)
  - Abscess (painful, hot & swollen breast)

3.2. Triple assessment of a breast lump
1. Clinical examination
2. Imaging (USS/mammography)
3. Fine needle aspiration

3.3. Breast dimpling
- Does not necessarily imply invasion of cancer into underlying musculature
- Intra-mammary tumour can pull on a Cooper ligament, causing dimpling of the skin
- The action of raising the hands above the head tends to accentuate this

4. Scrotal lump notes

4.1. DD Painless scrotal swelling (excludes inguinoscrotal hernia):

	Tumour	Hydrocoele	Epididymal cyst	Varicocoele
Characteristics	Firm mass	Soft & smooth (may be large)	Soft & smooth	'Bag of worms'
Relationship to testis	Continuous	Continuous	Separate	Separate
Transillumination	–	✓✓	✓	–
Other information	See below	May be due to underlying tumour Rarely congenital	Also known as spermatocoele	Examine SU standing (may disappear when supine) More common on left* [see notes 4.3] ↑ incidence of infertility Rarely due to renal Ca

4.2. DD Painful scrotal swelling
- Testicular torsion
- Torsion of testicular appendage
- Epididymo-orchitis
- Scrotal abscess
- Traumatic scrotal haematoma

4.3. Varicocoele more common on left side
- Right spermatic vein drains into IVC
  - Short, direct course
  - Lower incidence of valvular pathology
- Left spermatic vein drains into left renal vein
  - Long, tortuous course
  - Valves often absent or incompetent
  - Rarely, obstructed by renal Ca – new diagnosis of left varicocoele requires an abdominal USS to exclude

4.4. Testicular tumours
- Relatively rare but most common tumour in young & middle-aged men
- Presentation
  - Painless lump in testis
  - Testicular enlargement
  - Scrotal pain/dragging sensation
  - Gynaecomastia (if high β-hCG)

5. Hernia notes

5.1. Definition of a hernia

The protrusion of whole or part of a viscus through an opening in the wall of its containing cavity into a place where it is not normally found.

5.2. Complications of a hernia

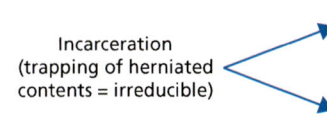

Incarceration (trapping of herniated contents = irreducible)

1. Obstruction (clinically: pain, constipation, vomiting, distension)

2. Strangulation -> ischaemia -> necrosis -> peritonitis

5.3. Risk factors for developing a hernia

- Family history
- Weakness of abdominal musculature
  - Increasing age (especially direct)
  - Surgery (incisional hernia)
- Increased intra-abdominal pressure
  - Obesity
  - Pregnancy
  - Other organomegaly
  - COPD/chronic cough
  - Prostatism
  - Constipation
  - Heavy lifting

5.4. Types of hernia

	Features	Surgical indications*
Indirect inguinal hernia	• Through inguinal ring, down inguinal canal & out of external ring • Superior to pubic tubercle • Commonly extends into scrotum • Can be very large • Reducible • Low risk of incarceration	Surgical repair recommended as impossible to detect if indirect on examination alone
Direct inguinal hernia	• Through weak point in Hesselbach's triangle • Superior to pubic tubercle • Rarely extends into scrotum • Almost always reducible • Low risk of incarceration	Surgical repair
Femoral	• Through femoral canal underneath inguinal ligament • Inferior to pubic tubercle • Never extends into scrotum • Rarely reducible • Usually incarcerated with high risk of strangulation	Urgent surgical repair
Para-umbilical (acquired)	• Through linea alba above umbilicus (rarely below) • Often reducible • High risk of incarceration	Surgical repair
True umbilical (congenital)	• Through umbilicus • Usually resolves spontaneously in early life	Surgical repair if persists >5 years of age
Epigastric	• Through linea alba in epigastrium • Low risk of incarceration (usually contains only fat)	Elective surgical repair recommended as most will enlarge
Spigelian	• Through linea semilunaris at outer border of rectus sheath • High risk of incarceration & strangulation	Urgent surgical repair
Incisional	• Can occur anywhere but especially midline surgery • Usually progressively enlarges • Usually reducible • Moderate risk of incarceration	Surgical repair for cosmetic reasons

* Most incarcerated & all strangulated hernias require urgent surgical repair.

APPENDIX: SKIN LESIONS

SKIN LESIONS

This sequence can be used for any skin lesion, including pigmented lesions, non-pigmented lesions & rashes. The examination should also include examination of regional lymph nodes [**see Appendix: Lymph nodes**].

! BEFORE starting the examination !

SU perspective: proactively explore any potential concerns beforehand

- Concern that a skin lesion could be cancer: explain the importance of moving through a series of checks together to help guide what to do next / who to refer to, to move forward with support
- Concern about appearance of lesion(s): acknowledge & reassure around the need for assessment to make an informed shared decision
- Concerns about being contagious to others: provide information about likelihood & how to minimise risk if present
- Concern for exposure: explain the extent of exposure required, reassure about maintaining dignity, & offer a chaperone

EXAMINATION OF A SKIN LESION

Component / action	Examine for	DD / potential findings / extra information
Use draping to expose only as required for each examination step **Inspection:** Distribution (of rash [**see notes 1**])	• Symmetrical	→ Systemic (endogenous) aetiology, e.g. atopic dermatitis, drug reaction, viral exanthems, erythema nodosum
	• Asymmetrical	→ External aetiology, e.g. infection, trauma, contact dermatitis
Shape/configuration	• Discrete	→ e.g. mole, seborrhoeic keratosis
	• Confluent	→ e.g. urticaria, measles rash
	• Linear	→ e.g. scabies burrow
	• Discoid	→ e.g. discoid eczema, discoid lupus erythematosus
	• Target	→ e.g. erythema multiforme, erythema migrans
	• Annular	→ e.g. tinea corporis
Colour	• Erythematous	→ e.g. cellulitis
	• Purpuric	→ e.g. meningococcal septicaemia, vasculitis
	• Hyperpigmented	→ e.g. melasma, Addison's disease
	• Hypopigmented	→ e.g. vitiligo, pityriasis versicolor
Border	• Regular	→ Likely benign, e.g. moles
	• Irregular	→ Suspicious of malignancy, e.g. melanoma [**see notes 2 & 3**]
Morphology	• [**see notes 4**]	→ [**see notes 4**]

APPENDIX: SKIN LESIONS

Palpation:		
Texture	• Smooth	→ e.g. ecchymoses, lichen planus, erythema nodosum
	• Rough	→ e.g. psoriasis, actinic keratosis
	• Crusty	→ e.g. impetigo, psoriasis
Elevation [see notes 4]	• Elevated (papule, plaque, nodule)	→ e.g. psoriasis, acne, naevi
	• Flat (macule, patch)	→ e.g. vitiligo, petechiae, melasma
Temperature	• Increased warmth	→ Infection (cellulitis), inflammation (urticaria), e.g. erythema nodosum [see notes 5]
Consistency	• Soft	→ e.g. cyst
	• Firm	→ e.g. dermatofibroma
	• Hard	→ e.g. malignancy, calcified lesions, chronic inflammation
Fluctuance	• Fluctuant	→ e.g. abscess, cyst, inflamed sebaceous cyst
Mobility	• Fixed	→ e.g. malignancy, deep infection, chronic inflammation with fibrosis
Tenderness	• Tender	→ e.g. infection, inflammation, rapidly growing tumour, erythema nodosum [see notes 5]
Blanching (apply light pressure)	• Blanching	→ e.g. erythema
Palpate regional lymph nodes [see **Appendix: Lymph nodes**]	• Non-blanching	→ e.g. purpura, erythema nodosum (see notes 5)
	• Lymphadenopathy	→ [see Appendix: Lymph nodes]

Examination of a skin lesion may then be followed by further tests to assist in making a diagnosis. These might include biopsy for histology, skin swabs or scraping for microbiology, dermoscopy to visualise pigment networks & vessels, patch tests to identify hypersensitivity reactions, Wood's light (long-range UVA) for pigmentary changes & fluorescence.

1. Distribution of a rash
- Acral – involving the extremities, especially hands, feet, fingers, toes (e.g. dyshidrotic eczema, hand, foot, & mouth disease)
- Extensor – involving the outer (extensor) surfaces of joints such as elbows & knees (e.g. psoriasis, lichen planus)
  Flexural – involving body folds or flexural surfaces, such as behind knees, elbows, groin, axillae (e.g. atopic dermatitis, candidiasis)
- Follicular – centred around hair follicles (e.g. folliculitis, acne vulgaris)
- Dermatomal – follows the distribution of a dermatome (e.g. herpes zoster, segmental vitiligo)
- Seborrhoeic – affects sebaceous areas, such as scalp, face (nasolabial folds), chest, upper back (e.g. acne, rosacea, seborrhoeic dermatitis)

2. Warning signs of melanoma

Inspection using ABCDE approach: **A**symmetry in the colour / marking / features of lesion: - **B**order - **C**olour - **D**iameter - **E**volution	- Irregular border - More than 2 colours - Larger than 6mm - Fast growing / changing in appearance

3. Weighted 7-point checklist for assessment of pigmented skin lesions
Use this weighted 7-point checklist for assessment of pigmented skin lesions & to determine the need for referral.
- Major features of the lesion (2 points each):
  - Change in size
  - Irregular shape
  - Irregular colour
- Minor features of the lesion (1 point each):
  - Largest diameter 7mm or more
  - Inflammation
  - Oozing
  - Change in sensation (including itch)

Referral using the urgent suspected cancer pathway should be made for a suspicious lesion with a weighted 7-point checklist score of 3 or more.

NOTES

4. Morphology: how to describe skin lesions

Lesion type	Description	Examples of skin conditions
Macule	Flat area of altered colour <1.5cm in diameter	Freckles (e.g. axillary in neurofibromatosis type 1), flat melanocytic naevus, petechiae, vitiligo (early)
Patch	Flat area of altered colour >1.5cm	Vitiligo, melasma, café-au-lait spots (neurofibromatosis type 1), pityriasis versicolor
Papule	Solid, raised, palpable lesion <0.5cm	Molluscum contagiosum, acne (closed comedones), lichen planus, warts, rosacea, neurofibromatosis type 1
Nodule	Solid, raised, palpable lesion >0.5cm	Dermatofibroma, lipoma, basal cell carcinoma (nodular type), rheumatoid nodules, erythema nodosum
Plaque	Palpable flat lesion >1cm, usually raised or thickened	Psoriasis, eczema (chronic), *Tinea corporis*, *Mycosis fungoides*
Vesicle	Raised, clear fluid-filled lesion <0.5cm	Chickenpox, herpes simplex, dyshidrotic eczema, hand foot & mouth disease
Bulla	Raised, clear fluid-filled lesion >0.5cm	Bullous pemphigoid, pemphigus vulgaris, insect bites, friction blister
Pustule	Pus-containing lesion <0.5cm	Acne vulgaris, folliculitis, impetigo, pustular psoriasis, rosacea
Abscess	Localised accumulation of pus (usually deep, tender, fluctuant)	Skin abscess, furuncle, hidradenitis suppurativa
Wheal	Oedematous papule or plaque (from dermal oedema), transient	Urticaria (hives), insect bites, dermatographism
Boil/furuncle	Painful *Staph.* infection of hair follicle, often with central necrosis	Furunculosis, infected folliculitis
Carbuncle	Group of infected adjacent follicles (multiple boils), often with systemic signs	Severe *Staph.* infections, diabetic skin infections

NOTES

5. DD Erythema nodosum

Erythema nodosum often appears in clinically significant settings like autoimmune disease, infection, or drug reaction, so it's important to recognise, especially when paired with systemic symptoms (fever, malaise, arthralgia).

- Painful, purple, raised lesions on shins
- Idiopathic (up to 55% of cases)
- Sarcoidosis (30–40% of cases)
- Infection:
  - Streptococci
  - TB
- IBD
- Drugs
  - OCP
  - Sulphonamides
- Malignancy
  - Lymphoma
  - Leukaemia
- Pregnancy

NOTES